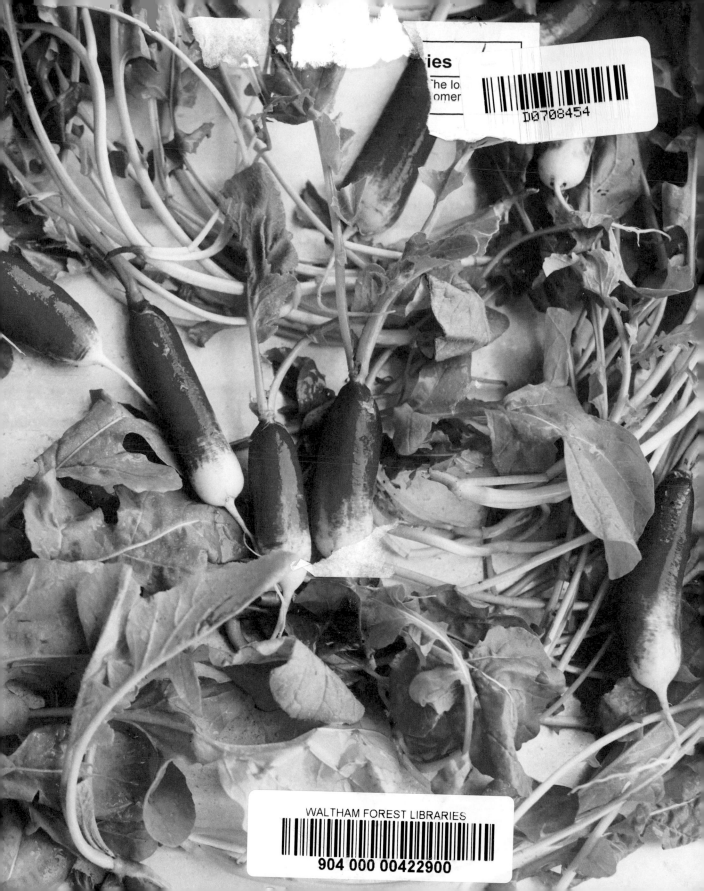

the salad bowl

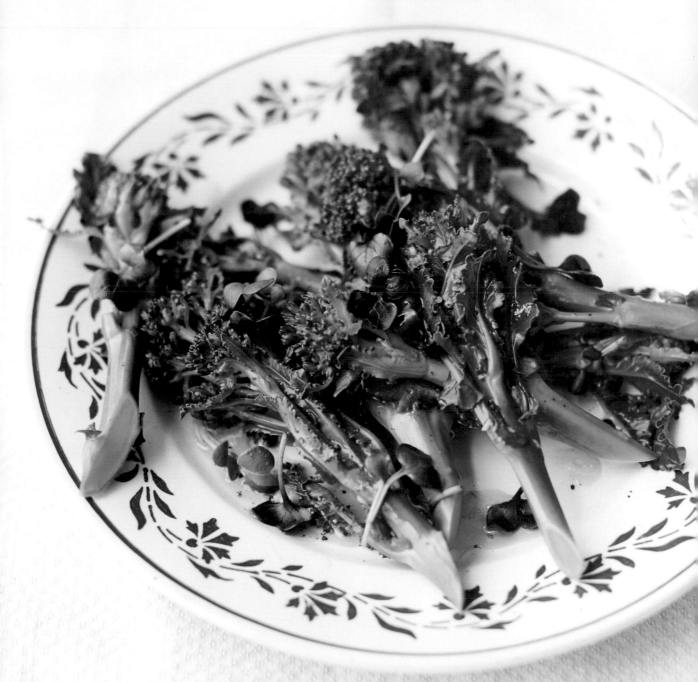

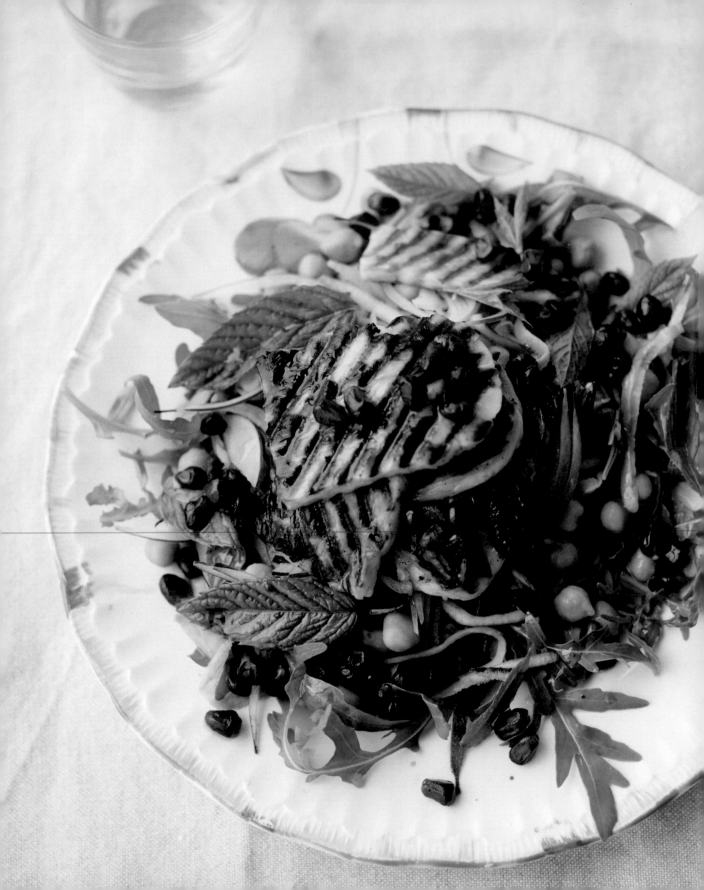

the
salad bowl

vibrant & healthy recipes
for light meals, lunches,
simple sides & dressings

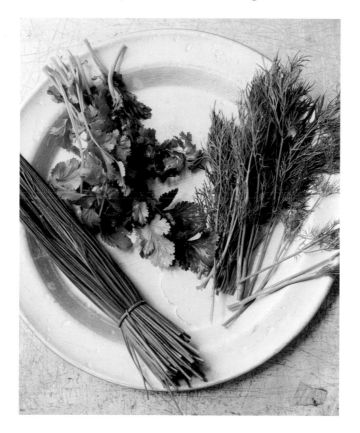

Nicola Graimes
photography by Matt Russell

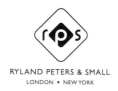

RYLAND PETERS & SMALL
LONDON • NEW YORK

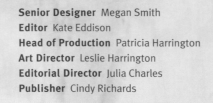

Senior Designer Megan Smith
Editor Kate Eddison
Head of Production Patricia Harrington
Art Director Leslie Harrington
Editorial Director Julia Charles
Publisher Cindy Richards

Prop Stylist Jo Harris
Food Stylist Aya Nishimura
Assistant Food Stylist Xenia Von Oswald
Indexer Hilary Bird

First published in 2015 by
Ryland Peters & Small
20–21 Jockey's Fields,
London WC1R 4BW
and
341 E 116th St
New York NY 10029
www.rylandpeters.com

Text © Nicola Graimes 2015
Design and photographs ©
Ryland Peters & Small 2015

ISBN: 978-1-84975-601-3

Printed and bound in China

10 9 8 7 6 5 4 3 2 1

NOTES

• Both British (Metric)
and American (Imperial plus
US cups) measurements
and ingredients are included
in these recipes for your
convenience, however it is
important to work with one
set of measurements and not
alternate between the two
within a recipe. Spellings
are primarily British.

• All spoon measurements
are level unless otherwise
specified.

• All eggs are medium (UK)
or large (US), unless specified
as large, in which case US
extra-large should be used.
Uncooked or partially cooked
eggs should not be served
to the very old, frail, young
children, pregnant women
or those with compromised
immune systems.

• When a recipe calls for the
grated zest of citrus fruit, buy
unwaxed fruit and wash well
before using. If you can only
find treated fruit, scrub well
in warm, soapy water and
rinse before using.

• Ovens should be preheated
to the specified temperatures.
We recommend using an
oven thermometer. If using
a fan-assisted oven, adjust
temperatures according to the
manufacturer's instructions.

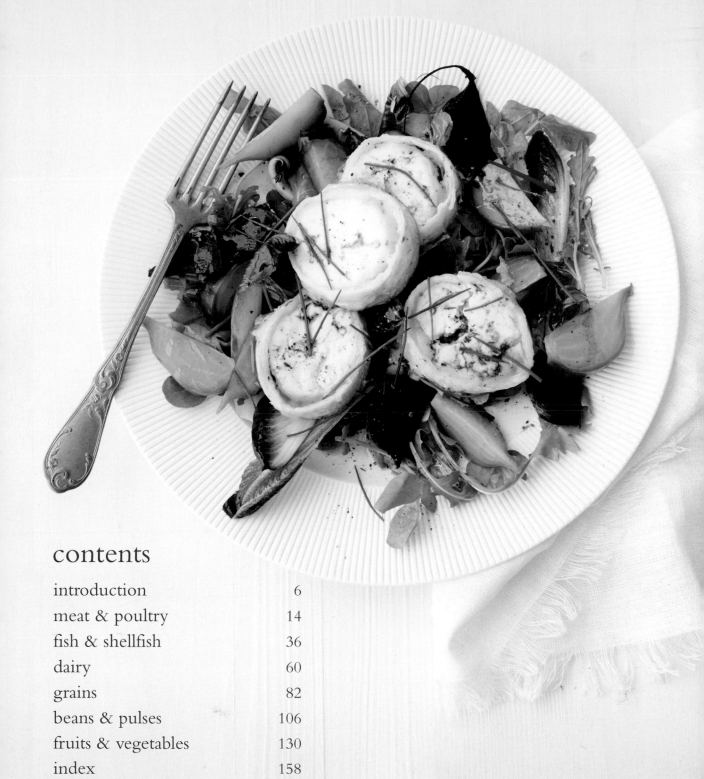

contents

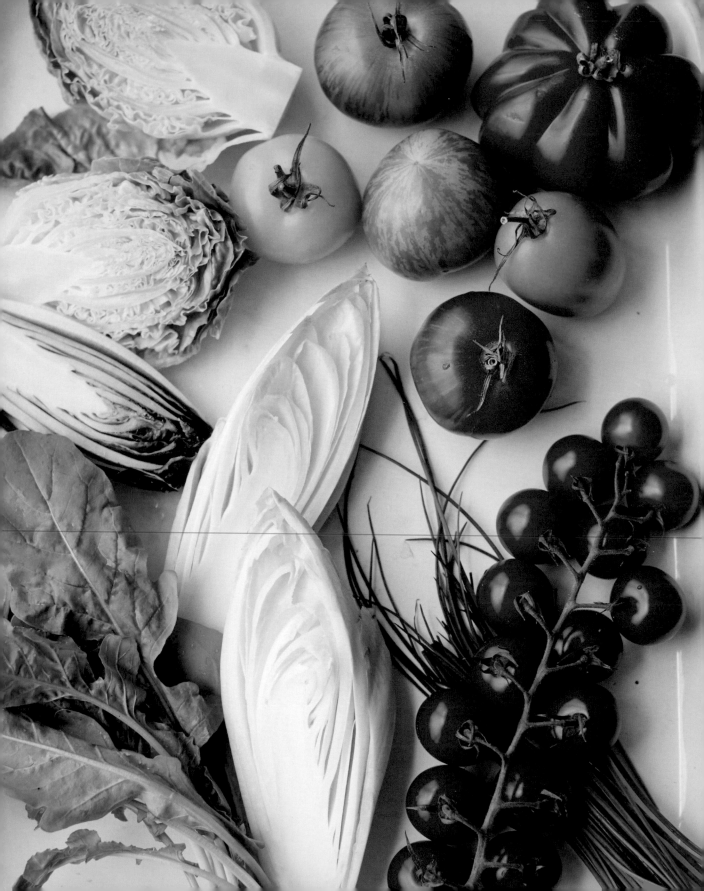

introduction

When you think of salad, lettuce immediately springs to mind, but happily the days are long gone when the most exotic salad leaf available to buy belonged to the crisp iceberg lettuce. Now we're spoilt for choice with leaves of all shapes, sizes, colours and textures, from peppery mizuna and bitter-tasting frisée to spicy watercress and lemony, sharp sorrel. Yet salad now refers to so much more than a humble bowlful of lettuce leaves. As well as salads made principally from fresh fruit and vegetables, the book features a wealth of recipes that include grains, beans, pulses, dairy, meat, poultry, fish and shellfish.

Making a good salad is totally dependent on the quality of ingredients you use. If feasible, choose local and seasonal fresh produce – organic is even better. Wilted, damaged leaves and vegetables will obviously result in a lacklustre salad, which is deficient in nutritional value. Similarly, choose loose fresh produce over packaged, that way you can inspect what you are buying. Bagged salad leaves are often washed in chlorine before being packed and can be expensive to buy.

A salad of soft, mild butterhead lettuce dressed simply in extra virgin olive oil and a sprinkling of sea salt, and perhaps a squeeze of lemon juice, is a simple pleasure. However, when the occasion arises, it's good to step it up a gear and experiment with various types of salad leaves concentrating on offering a range of textures, tastes and colours. A sprinkling of fresh herbs and flowers, including marigolds, nasturtiums, violets, chives and wild garlic, add a visual and flavour boost.

Tomatoes (opt for vine-ripened and in-season for the best flavour) and cucumber are classic additions to a salad, but there is a wealth of other fresh produce to try. Instead of cooking courgettes/zucchini, cauliflower, broccoli, cabbage, kale, beetroot/beets, asparagus and peas, try them raw in a salad.

Consider growing your own salad leaves (or other veg); you don't even need a garden! A few cut-and-come-again lettuce seeds sprinkled into a windowbox, pot, or grow-bag will provide you with a steady supply of leaves throughout the summer. Rather than harvest the whole lettuce, just pick the outer leaves and the plant will provide you with new leaves. Rocket/arugula, mizuna, mustard leaves, spinach and loose-leaf lettuces are all easy to grow. It's feasible to sow seeds in the autumn for a supply of leaves through the winter months. It's not only immensely satisfying to grow your own fresh produce, but more economical, too.

Foraged leaves, such as young nettles, watercress, dandelions, rocket/arugula, sorrel, fat hen, sea beet or wild spinach, samphire and wild garlic, as well as wild fresh herbs, including oregano, marjoram and thyme all add extra interest and are fun to discover.

Salads aren't just for the warmer times of the year. A leafy salad makes an ideal palate cleanser following a substantial or rich meal, while warm salads are perfect for the winter months. Roasted vegetables dressed in a robust dressing of red wine vinegar, wholegrain mustard and maple syrup or with a drizzle of rosemary oil and roasted garlic are perfect served warm or at room temperature. Grains, beans and lentils all make satisfying salads and are ideal for when it's cold outside and for transforming a side dish into a main meal. Puy and green lentils hold their shape when cooked, while quinoa, couscous, barley, bulghur wheat, freekeh and kamut are all worth checking out, as they add texture as well as nutrients. It often pays to cook more than you need for an evening meal to use the following day in a lunch.

Leftover cooked potatoes, pasta, rice, meats or salmon are all welcome additions to a salad. Choose a dressing to complement the ingredients and you've given a new lease of life to leftovers. Protein-rich nuts, seeds, cheese, meat, poultry, fish, shellfish, beans, lentils, some grains, tofu and eggs are a welcome source of nutrients in salads. Fresh and dried fruit, especially apricots, figs, raisins, soured cherries and cranberries, add vitamins, minerals and fibre to salads, as well as countering any bitterness with their natural sweetness. Choose fresh fruit in season and at the peak of ripeness.

The recipes is this book will hopefully show that there is a wealth of ways to make interesting, healthy, delicious salads. Using a little imagination and creativity the possibilities for feel-good food are almost endless.

preparing salads

The beauty of salads are that they are simple to prepare and don't require expensive cookware. There are some basic rules on washing and dressing salads and a few kitchen tools that can make life easier, but a good, sharp knife and a chopping board are the only essentials.

Washing salad leaves

Even if your bag of salad says "ready-to-eat" or "ready-washed" on the label, it's best to wash the contents to get rid of any chemical additives, as well as bugs or other possible contaminants. Gently wash them in a sink of cold water, separating the leaves first, if necessary. Drain the leaves and gently dry them in a salad spinner, taking care not to bruise them.

Dressing salads

Salad leaves are best dressed just before serving to prevent them going soggy. Be careful not to use too much dressing; you need just enough to lightly coat. Toss gently with your hands or tongs to combine. Conversely, grain, bean and lentil salads are best dressed in advance to allow the flavours to develop. Avocados, apples and pears benefit from a squeeze of lemon juice to stop them discolouring when the cut surface is exposed to air.

Useful salad tools

A few basic, everyday kitchen tools will help you create a variety of salads at home. There's nothing fancy in the list and, in fact, they are pretty much all kitchen staples.

Knives: buy the best you can afford and sharpen them regularly to keep in peak condition and then you'll be rewarded with a set of knifes that will last for years. A basic set includes a cook's knife; fruit or vegetable paring knife; filleting knife; bread knife; carving knife and a serrated fruit or vegetable knife.

Chopping boards: have separate chopping boards for raw meat, cooked food and strong foods such as onions and garlic, which can taint a board.

Salad spinner: this makes easy work of drying salad leaves without damaging them.

Vegetable peeler: not only good for peeling fruit and vegetables, you can also use it to slice Parmesan into shavings as well as cut cucumber, courgettes/zucchini and carrots into ribbons.

Other tools: box grater; storage jars; a small hand whisk; storage boxes; scissors; and a pestle and mortar.

Non-essential tools

Mandoline: perfect for cutting vegetables into various thicknesses and shapes, including paper-thin slices and crinkle cut chips. Make sure your mandoline is sturdy with a protective hand guard.

Spiralizer: popular in raw food circles, the spiralizer makes easy work of cutting vegetables into "spaghetti", "noodles", thin ribbons and attractive spiral strands.

Sprout germinator: seed germinators come in many shapes and sizes and while a large jam jar will suffice (see below), regular sprouters may like to invest in a larger germinator with stacking trays. It not only allows you to sow different varieties of seed at a time, but aids air circulation, light accessibility and rinsing.

Sprouting

Beans, lentils, grains and seeds can all be sprouted or germinated, a simple process that increases their nutritional value as well as increasing their digestibility. For instance, there is around 60 per cent more vitamin C and 30 per cent more B vitamins in the sprouted bean or grain than the unsprouted. Sprouts of various types are increasingly available in supermarkets and health foods stores, but DIY sprouting is also very easy to do at home and there are numerous seeds now available to buy.

   If you sprout regularly, then it may be worth investing in a sprout germinator (see above). Alternatively, a jam jar, a small piece of muslin/cheesecloth and an elastic band are all you need. The method is exactly the same for all grains, beans, lentils and seeds; it's simply the germination time that varies, ranging from 1–4 days. Large beans, such as chickpeas and wholegrains including wheatberries, take longer than the smaller alfalfa or amaranth seeds.

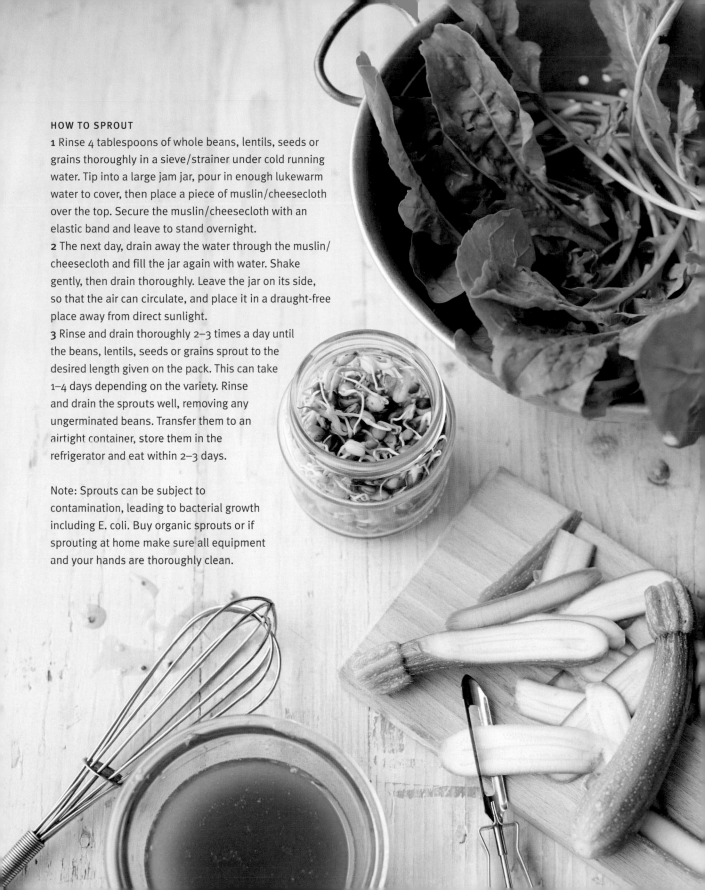

HOW TO SPROUT

1 Rinse 4 tablespoons of whole beans, lentils, seeds or grains thoroughly in a sieve/strainer under cold running water. Tip into a large jam jar, pour in enough lukewarm water to cover, then place a piece of muslin/cheesecloth over the top. Secure the muslin/cheesecloth with an elastic band and leave to stand overnight.

2 The next day, drain away the water through the muslin/cheesecloth and fill the jar again with water. Shake gently, then drain thoroughly. Leave the jar on its side, so that the air can circulate, and place it in a draught-free place away from direct sunlight.

3 Rinse and drain thoroughly 2–3 times a day until the beans, lentils, seeds or grains sprout to the desired length given on the pack. This can take 1–4 days depending on the variety. Rinse and drain the sprouts well, removing any ungerminated beans. Transfer them to an airtight container, store them in the refrigerator and eat within 2–3 days.

Note: Sprouts can be subject to contamination, leading to bacterial growth including E. coli. Buy organic sprouts or if sprouting at home make sure all equipment and your hands are thoroughly clean.

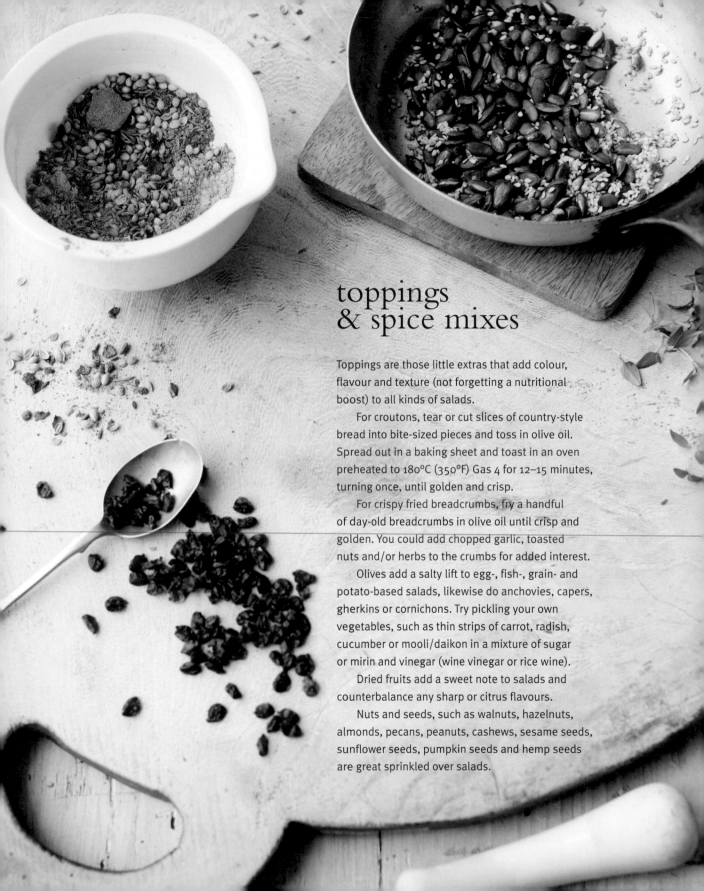

toppings & spice mixes

Toppings are those little extras that add colour, flavour and texture (not forgetting a nutritional boost) to all kinds of salads.

For croutons, tear or cut slices of country-style bread into bite-sized pieces and toss in olive oil. Spread out in a baking sheet and toast in an oven preheated to 180°C (350°F) Gas 4 for 12–15 minutes, turning once, until golden and crisp.

For crispy fried breadcrumbs, fry a handful of day-old breadcrumbs in olive oil until crisp and golden. You could add chopped garlic, toasted nuts and/or herbs to the crumbs for added interest.

Olives add a salty lift to egg-, fish-, grain- and potato-based salads, likewise do anchovies, capers, gherkins or cornichons. Try pickling your own vegetables, such as thin strips of carrot, radish, cucumber or mooli/daikon in a mixture of sugar or mirin and vinegar (wine vinegar or rice wine).

Dried fruits add a sweet note to salads and counterbalance any sharp or citrus flavours.

Nuts and seeds, such as walnuts, hazelnuts, almonds, pecans, peanuts, cashews, sesame seeds, sunflower seeds, pumpkin seeds and hemp seeds are great sprinkled over salads.

Roasting nuts and seeds

A light toasting enhances the flavour of nuts and seeds and gives them extra crunch, but keep an eye on them as they can easily burn. Oven roasting is preferable for a large quantity, as it gives a more even roasting and colour, but it is less economical for small quantities unless you are using the oven to cook something else.

TO OVEN ROAST

Preheat the oven to 180°C (350°F) Gas 4. Line 1–2 baking sheets with baking parchment and sprinkle over the nuts (or seeds) in an even layer. Roast for 12–15 minutes, depending on their size, turning once, until light golden all over. Remove from the oven and let cool.

TO PAN ROAST

Sprinkle the nuts (or seeds) over the bottom of a large, dry frying pan/skillet in an even layer. Toast over a medium-low heat for 8–10 minutes for nuts; 5–7 minutes for large seeds; and 3–4 minutes for small seeds, until lightly coloured (shake the pan often or turn large nuts). Let cool.

Spice Mixes

Whether sprinkled over the top or added to the dressing, spice mixes add oomph to salads. Store any unused spice mix in an airtight jar or container, for a few weeks.

ZA'ATAR

The recipe for this popular Middle Eastern spice blend varies from country to cook, but is based on sumac, a citrusy red spice. Don't limit za'atar to salads; it can also be sprinkled over eggs, yogurt-based dips or hummus, or used as a rub for meat or fish.

3 tablespoons thyme leaves (or 1½ tablespoons dried)
2 teaspoons sumac
½ teaspoon sea salt
1 tablespoon sesame seeds, toasted

Preheat the oven to 160°C (325°F) Gas 3. Put the thyme on a small baking sheet in the oven for 5 minutes, or until dried. Crumble the thyme leaves into a bowl and mix in the sumac, salt and sesame seeds. Let cool and transfer to an airtight container if not using immediately.

CHAAT MASALA

This popular Indian spice mix adds a kick to potato, bean and lentil salads, as well as yogurt dressings. Dried mango (amchoor) powder is a must and can be found in Asian grocers, but you can be flexible with the other spices.

1 tablespoon cumin seeds
1 tablespoon coriander seeds
2 teaspoons dried mango (amchoor) powder
2 teaspoons garam masala
½ teaspoon dried chilli flakes/hot pepper flakes
1 teaspoon ground ginger
½ teaspoon sea salt
¼ teaspoon freshly ground black pepper

Toast the cumin and coriander seeds in a dry frying pan/skillet over a low heat for 2–3 minutes, or until aromatic. Using a pestle and mortar, grind the seeds to a powder, then stir in the remaining ingredients until combined.

DUKKAH

This Egyptian blend of spices, nuts and seeds is typically stirred into olive oil to make a dip for flatbreads, but it is also good sprinkled over a tomato salad with a splash of olive oil or stirred into grain- or lentil-based salads.

3 tablespoons coriander seeds
2 teaspoons cumin seeds
2 tablespoons sesame seeds
3 tablespoons sunflower seeds
3 tablespoons pumpkin seeds
40 g/⅓ cup hazelnuts
40 g/⅓ cup blanched almonds
½ teaspoon dried chilli/hot pepper flakes
sea salt and freshly ground black pepper

Put all the seeds in a dry frying pan/skillet and toast for 2–3 minutes, shaking the pan occasionally, until they are aromatic and start to colour. Tip out of the pan and let cool.

Next, add the nuts to the pan and cook for 5 minutes, shaking the pan occasionally, until they smell toasted and start to colour. Tip out of the pan and let cool.

Put the toasted seeds and nuts in a mini grinder and grind to a coarse, crumbly mixture. Transfer to a bowl, stir in the dried chilli/hot pepper flakes and season well.

dressings

A dressing brings a salad to life. It should complement, enhance and enliven your salad, rather than mask or confuse. Dressings can be as simple as a drizzle of extra virgin olive oil, a squeeze of lemon juice and a little seasoning, or more complex incorporating speciality nut oils or flavourings.

Although there are lots of different dressings, this book focuses on three main types: oil-based, such as a classic vinaigrette; creamy, such as mayonnaise-, cream- or crème fraîche-based; and non-oil, which includes Asian dressings that are based on rice vinegar, mirin or soy sauce.

Just as the quality of ingredients is vital for the best-tasting salad, so is the quality of the oils and vinegars you use. Go for the best you can afford and reserve them for salads, rather than for cooking.

When buying olive oil for salad dressings, opt for a first-pressed extra virgin oil. Try to buy oils from the current year's harvest and in dark, rather than clear, bottles as they are protected against the damaging effects of light.

Try experimenting with nut and seed oils (walnut, hazelnut, pistachio, pumpkin seed and sesame are all excellent), but be mindful of buying too many different varieties at once, as they have a limited shelf-life. Nut oils can also be quite strong in flavour, so are best used judiciously.

Similarly, there are a multitude of different vinegars and, as with oils, you should go for quality – the best wine vinegars are wood-aged. Opt for a selection, including a white wine vinegar, red wine vinegar, balsamic vinegar, sherry vinegar and rice vinegar.

Experimenting with different spices and herbs (either fresh or dried) can give a new lease of life to everyday salad dressings, as well as alter the feel of their culinary influence. For instance, spices such as cumin, coriander, chilli/chili powder and spice blends, including harissa and ras el hanout, lend a North African or Middle Eastern taste to salad dressings, while ginger, mustard seeds, onion seeds and garam masala are undoubtedly Indian.

Mayonnaise

Homemade mayonnaise is really satisfying to make and bears little resemblance to store-bought versions. Remember to add the oil very gradually in a slow, steady stream to prevent the mayonnaise curdling or separating. Use a good-quality, mild-flavoured oil, such as groundnut/ peanut or sunflower; extra virgin olive oil is too overpowering. You can make mayonnaise in a blender, but a hand whisk is just as effective for moderate amounts.

1 UK large/US extra large egg yolk
1 teaspoon Dijon mustard
150 ml/⅔ cup groundnut/peanut oil or sunflower oil
1 teaspoon white wine vinegar
a large pinch of sea salt and freshly ground black pepper
MAKES ABOUT 150 ML/⅔ CUP

1 Crack the egg into a mixing bowl. Whisk in the mustard and the salt and pepper until combined.
2 Holding the jug of oil in one hand and the whisk in the other, pour in a drop of oil and whisk in. Continue to add the oil a drop at a time until the mixture starts to thicken, then slowly pour in the remaining oil in a steady stream, whisking continuously, until the mixture becomes opaque and thickens to a smooth, glossy sauce. (If the mayonnaise curdles, you can reclaim it by very gradually adding the curdled mixture to a second egg yolk and mustard mixture, initially a drop at a time. Continue adding the oil until smooth, thickened and creamy.)
3 Whisk in the vinegar to taste and add more salt and pepper if needed. Store in a screw-top jar in the refrigerator for up to 1 week.

VARIATIONS
• Stir in 1 crushed small clove garlic to make alioli.
• Stir in 2 tablespoons horseradish or tartare sauce and 1 teaspoon chopped capers.
• Stir in 1 tablespoon sweet chilli/chili sauce or 1 teaspoon harissa paste and a squeeze of lemon juice.
• Stir in the juice of ½ lemon instead of the vinegar along with 4 tablespoons chopped fresh herbs such as chives, dill, oregano, parsley or basil, or a combination.

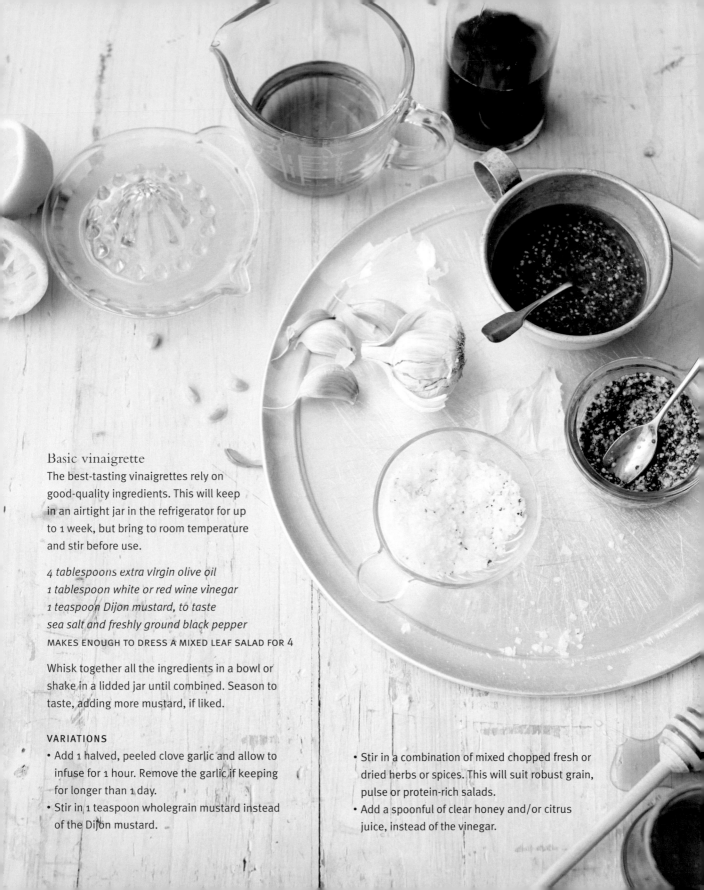

Basic vinaigrette

The best-tasting vinaigrettes rely on
good-quality ingredients. This will keep
in an airtight jar in the refrigerator for up
to 1 week, but bring to room temperature
and stir before use.

4 tablespoons extra virgin olive oil
1 tablespoon white or red wine vinegar
1 teaspoon Dijon mustard, to taste
sea salt and freshly ground black pepper
MAKES ENOUGH TO DRESS A MIXED LEAF SALAD FOR 4

Whisk together all the ingredients in a bowl or
shake in a lidded jar until combined. Season to
taste, adding more mustard, if liked.

VARIATIONS

• Add 1 halved, peeled clove garlic and allow to
  infuse for 1 hour. Remove the garlic if keeping
  for longer than 1 day.
• Stir in 1 teaspoon wholegrain mustard instead
  of the Dijon mustard.

• Stir in a combination of mixed chopped fresh or
  dried herbs or spices. This will suit robust grain,
  pulse or protein-rich salads.
• Add a spoonful of clear honey and/or citrus
  juice, instead of the vinegar.

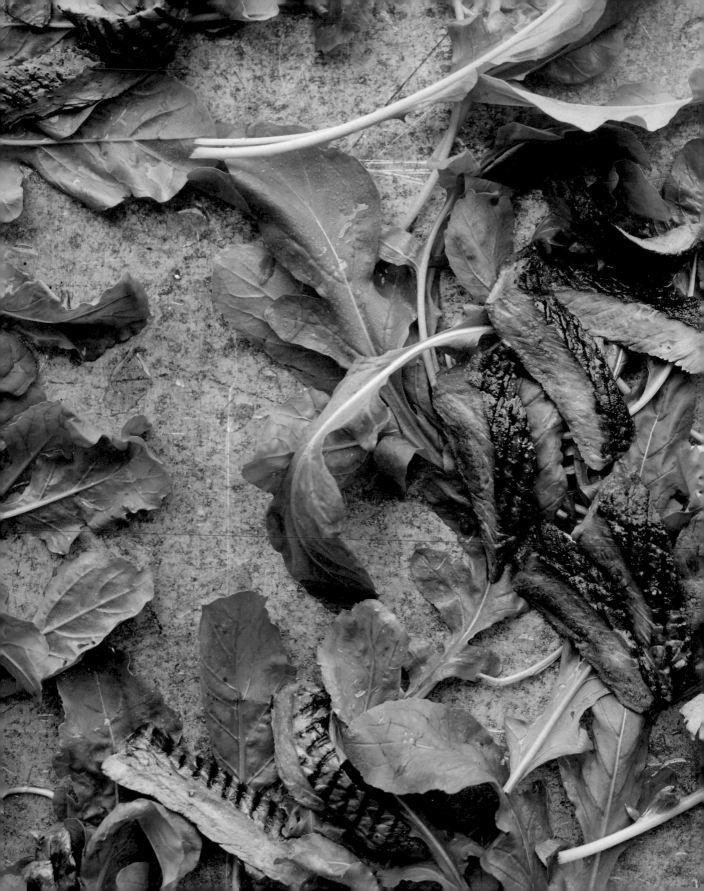

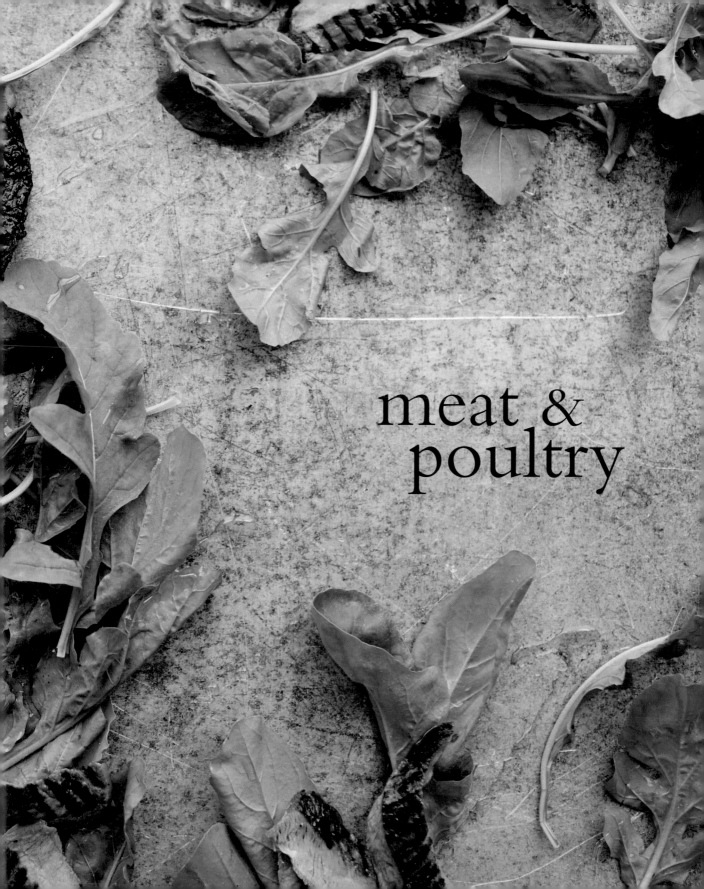

meat &
poultry

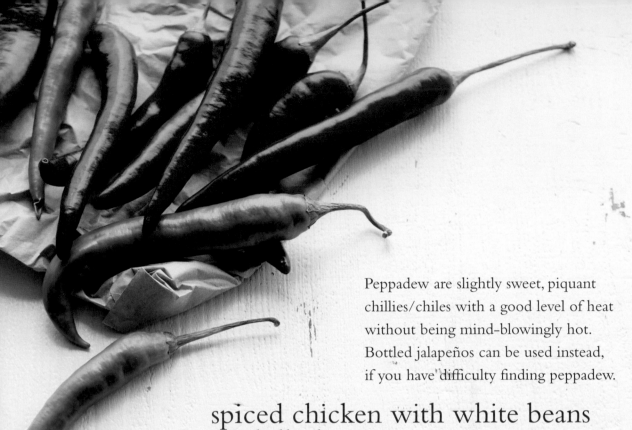

Peppadew are slightly sweet, piquant chillies/chiles with a good level of heat without being mind-blowingly hot. Bottled jalapeños can be used instead, if you have difficulty finding peppadew.

spiced chicken with white beans & chilli dressing

3 skinless, boneless chicken breasts

1 tablespoon smoked paprika

1 tablespoon olive oil

1 large yellow (bell) pepper, seeded and thinly sliced

300 g/11 oz. canned drained haricot/navy beans, rinsed

200 g/7 oz. vine-ripened cherry tomatoes, halved

1 banana shallot, thinly sliced

2 handfuls of basil leaves, torn

2 handfuls of coriander/ cilantro leaves

1 pitta bread, toasted until crisp and torn into pieces

CHILLI DRESSING

5 tablespoons extra virgin olive oil

freshly squeezed juice of 1½–2 limes, depending on how juicy they are

2 peppadew chillies in vinegar, drained and finely chopped

½ teaspoon dried chilli flakes/hot pepper flakes

sea salt and freshly ground black pepper

Serves 4

Put the chicken breasts between 2 sheets of clingfilm/ plastic wrap and flatten with a meat tenderizer or the end of a rolling pin until they are an even thickness, about 1.5 cm/½ in. Mix together the paprika with 1 tablespoon of the oil in a large, shallow dish. Season, add the chicken and spoon the marinade over the top until evenly coated.

Heat a ridged griddle pan over a high heat until hot. Turn the heat down slightly and char-grill the chicken in two batches for 7–10 minutes, turning twice, until cooked through and blackened in places. Leave to rest and cool slightly for 5 minutes, then slice into strips.

Meanwhile, to make the dressing, mix all the ingredients together in a bowl. Taste and add the extra lime juice, if needed. Season and set aside.

Put the (bell) pepper, beans, tomatoes, shallot and half the herbs in a large, shallow bowl. Spoon over half of the dressing and toss to coat everything. Top the salad with the chicken, remaining herbs and crisp pitta pieces and spoon over the rest of the dressing.

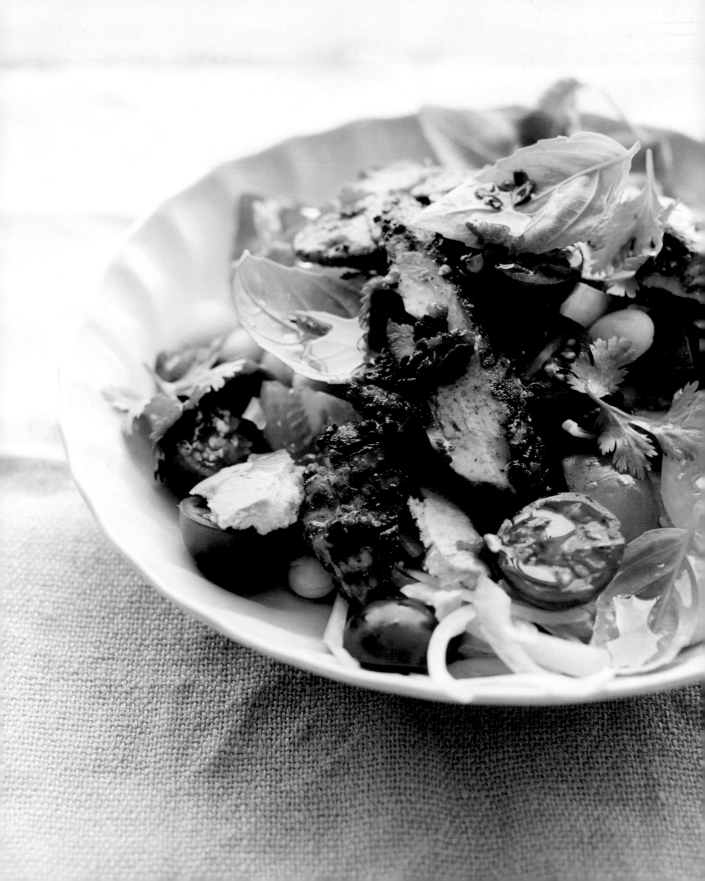

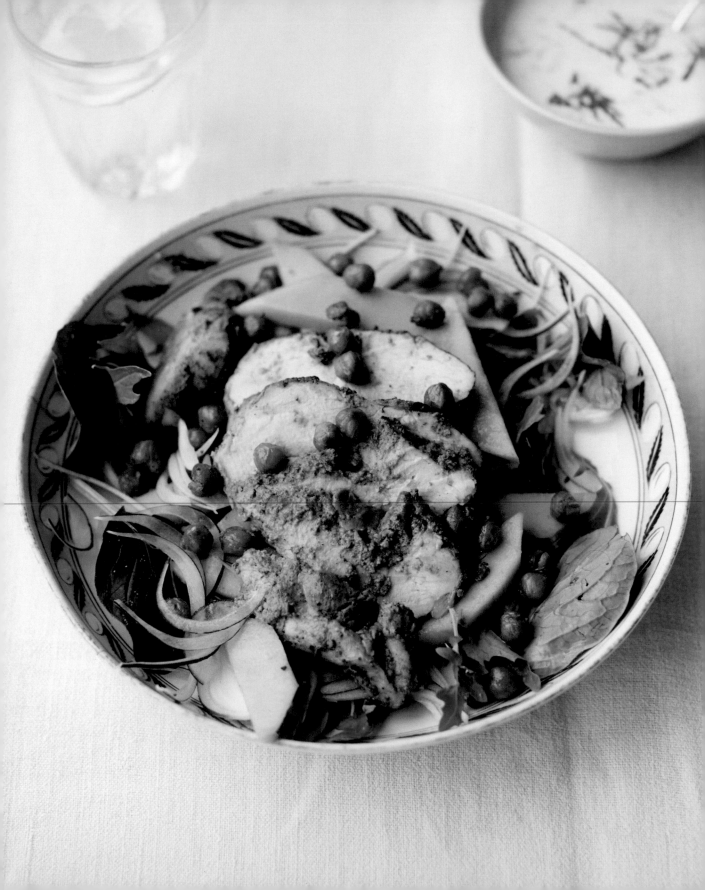

The combination of succulent spice-coated chicken, crisp roasted chickpeas and sweet, ripe mango is a real winner in this substantial salad. Serve with warm naan bread or roasted new potatoes.

tandoori chicken salad with crisp chickpeas & mango

1 heaped tablespoon
  tandoori spice mix
1 teaspoon turmeric
2 teaspoons garam
  masala
1 tablespoon sunflower
  oil, plus extra for
  drizzling
250 ml/generous 1 cup
  natural/plain yogurt
freshly squeezed juice
  of 1 large lemon
600 g/1lb 5oz. skinless,
  boneless chicken
  breasts
150 g/5½ oz. canned
  chickpeas, drained
4 heaped tablespoons
  freshly chopped mint
  leaves
4 large handfuls of
  mixed salad leaves
1 small red onion,
  cut into thin rings
1 mango, halved,
  stoned/pitted,
  peeled and sliced
sea salt and freshly
  ground black pepper

Serves 4

To make the marinade, mix together the tandoori spice mix, turmeric and garam masala in a large, shallow dish. Stir in the sunflower oil, 100 ml/scant ½ cup of the yogurt and half the lemon juice, and season. Add the chicken and spoon the marinade over until it is thoroughly coated, then leave to marinate for at least 30 minutes.

Preheat the oven to 200°C (400°F) Gas 6.

Put the chickpeas in a baking dish, drizzle over a little oil, season, and toss until they are coated. Roast in the preheated oven for 30 minutes, turning once, or until crisp and golden.

Meanwhile, put the chicken in a roasting pan, spoon any leftover marinade over and roast for 20–25 minutes, until cooked through and there is no trace of pink inside. Let the chicken rest for 5 minutes.

Mix together the remaining yogurt and lemon juice, season, then stir in the mint and 1 tablespoon water to make the dressing. Arrange the salad leaves on 4 serving plates and top with the onion and mango.

Cut the chicken diagonally into thin slices. Arrange the chicken pieces on top of the salad, drizzle the dressing on top and sprinkle with the crisp chickpeas.

CHICKEN

A marinade is the perfect way to add flavour to chicken as well as keep it moist during roasting. Seek out free-range, or preferably organic, poultry for the best flavour; it may be pricey, but it is well worth the extra cost.

Yuzu is a type of citrus fruit from Asia that is particularly popular in Japanese cooking. While it's difficult to find the fruit outside of Japan, it is now possible to buy bottles of the juice. It has an intense, tart, lemony flavour that cuts through the richness of the duck in this salad.

duck salad with yuzu dressing

2 tablespoons light
  soy sauce
1 tablespoon sesame oil
350 g/12 oz. duck breast
  mini-fillets
100 g/3¾ oz. watercress
  or rocket/arugula
  leaves
60 g/2 oz. Ruby Gem/
  Bibb lettuce or similar
  red leaf salad, sliced
60 g/2 oz. sugar snap
  peas, sliced diagonally
100 g/3¾ oz. radishes,
  sliced into rounds
2 handfuls of
  beansprouts
2 teaspoons toasted
  sesame seeds
2 spring onions/
  scallions, thinly sliced
  diagonally

YUZU DRESSING
2 tablespoons yuzu
  or lemon juice
6 tablespoons freshly
  squeezed orange juice
1 teaspoon ground ginger
2 teaspoons caster/
  superfine sugar
sea salt and freshly
  ground black pepper

Serves 4

Mix together the soy sauce and sesame oil in a dish. Add the duck and turn to coat in the marinade. Set aside for 15 minutes.

Meanwhile, to make the yuzu dressing, mix the yuzu, orange juice and ginger together. Stir in the caster/superfine sugar until it dissolves, and season to taste.

Combine the watercress, Ruby Gem/Bibb lettuce, sugar snap peas, radishes and beansprouts in a shallow serving bowl.

Heat a large, dry frying pan/skillet over a high heat, and when hot, add the duck and its marinade to the pan. Cook, turning the duck regularly, for 4–5 minutes, until it is cooked yet still slightly pink inside. Transfer the duck and any juices onto a plate and leave to rest for 5 minutes.

Arrange the duck on top of the salad and spoon enough of the dressing over to coat. Sprinkle with the sesame seeds and spring onions/scallions.

SUGAR SNAP PEAS
Sweet and crunchy, sugar snap peas (also known as snap peas) are just as delicious, if not more so, served raw in a salad as they are lightly steamed or stir-fried. Visually, they look pretty sliced on the diagonal so the peas inside the pod are exposed.

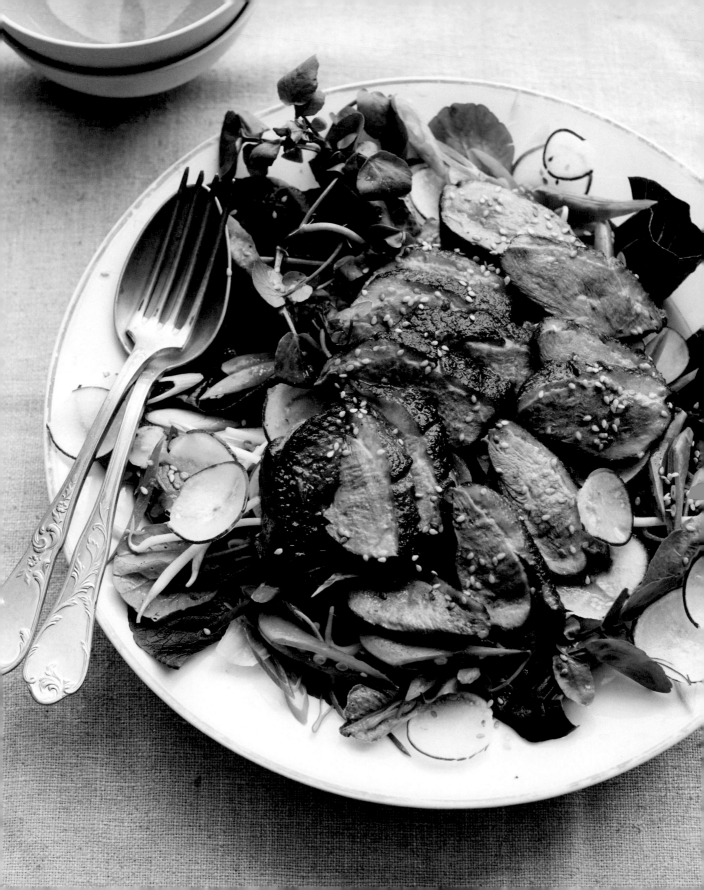

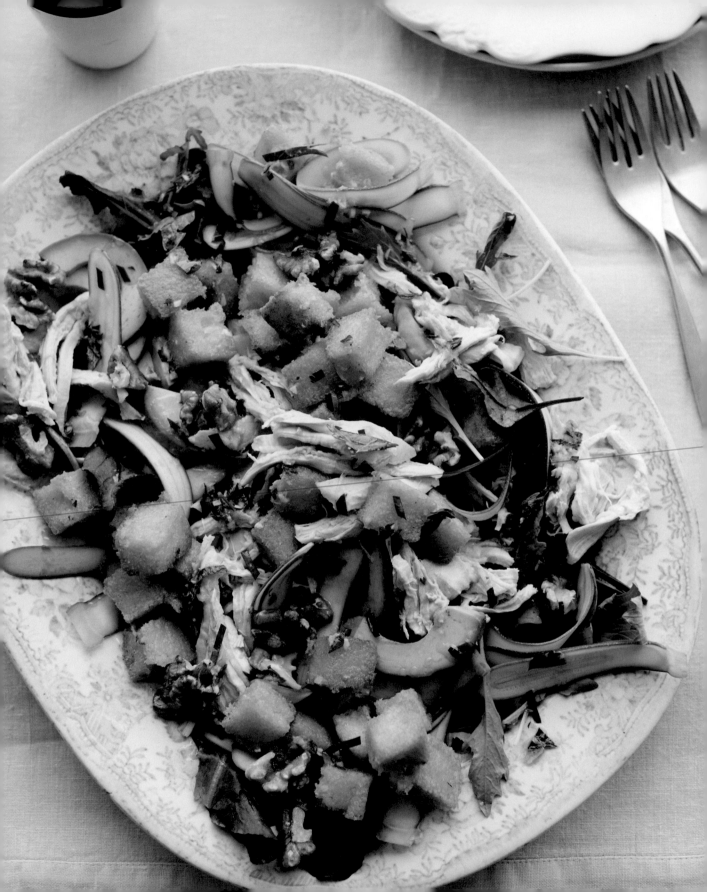

Although gremolata – the classic Italian mix of lemon, parsley and garlic – is most often used as a condiment or relish, with the addition of a fruity extra virgin olive oil, it makes a bright, fresh, flavour-packed dressing for a simple chicken salad.

roast chicken salad with gremolata & polenta croutons

2 tablespoons olive oil

300 g/11 oz. ready-cooked polenta, sliced and cut into croutons

140 g/4¾ oz. mixed soft salad leaves, including red leaves

300 g/11 oz. cooked roast chicken, shredded into long pieces

2 small avocados, peeled, halved, stoned/pitted and sliced

6 baby courgettes/zucchini, sliced into ribbons

50 g/½ cup walnut pieces, toasted

GREMOLATA DRESSING

5 tablespoons extra virgin olive oil

finely grated zest and freshly squeezed juice of 1 lemon

1 garlic clove, crushed

4 tablespoons finely chopped flat leaf parsley

sea salt and freshly ground black pepper

Serves 4

Heat the 2 tablespoons oil in a large, non-stick frying pan/skillet over a medium-high heat and fry the croutons for 10 minutes, turning occasionally, until crisp all over. Put the croutons on paper towels to remove any excess oil.

Meanwhile, mix together all the ingredients for the gremolata dressing and season to taste.

Arrange the salad leaves on a serving plate and top with the chicken, avocados and courgettes/zucchini. Spoon enough of the dressing over to lightly coat and toss gently, then sprinkle over the walnuts.

POLENTA

You could use a block of ready-made polenta to make the croutons for this recipe, but instant polenta or cornmeal takes a mere 5–10 minutes to make and has a superior flavour and texture. Follow the instructions on the pack, then spread out evenly on a greased baking sheet, about 1cm/½ in. thick, and leave to set – this doesn't take long. Cut into croutons and you're ready to go.

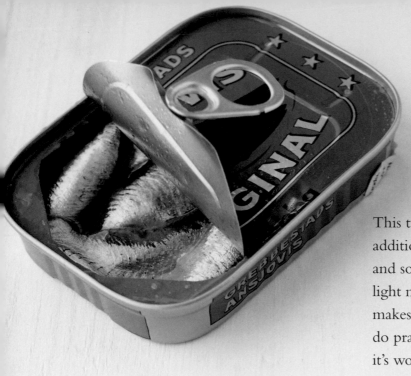

This twist on the original, with the addition of crisp shards of bacon, avocado and soft-boiled eggs makes a substantial light meal. Char-grilled chicken breast also makes a tasty alternative to the eggs, as do prawns/shrimp or canned tuna, so it's worth experimenting with your favourite additions.

crispy bacon Caesar salad

8 rashers/strips streaky/fatty bacon

4 thick slices ciabatta, torn into rough bite-sized croutons

2 tablespoons olive oil

8 large romaine or cos lettuce leaves, roughly torn

1 large avocado, peeled, halved, stoned/pitted and sliced

4 UK large/US extra-large soft-boiled/soft-cooked eggs, peeled and halved

DRESSING

3–4 anchovy fillets in oil, depending on their size, drained and sliced

3 tablespoons extra virgin olive oil

2 tablespoons mayonnaise (see recipe, page 12)

1 small garlic clove, crushed

freshly squeezed juice of ½ lemon, plus extra for squeezing over the avocado

½ teaspoon Dijon mustard

4 tablespoons finely grated Parmesan cheese

Serves 4

Preheat the oven to 200°C (400°F) Gas 6. Put the bacon in a roasting pan lined with foil and cook in the preheated oven for 15–20 minutes, turning once, or until crisp and golden. Drain the bacon on paper towels.

Meanwhile, put the croutons in a polythene food bag and add the oil. Shake the bag until the croutons are coated. Spread the croutons out evenly in a large roasting pan and toast in the oven for 10–15 minutes, turning once, until golden and crisp.

To make the dressing, blend all the ingredients in a blender until smooth and creamy, adding a little water if it is too thick; it should be the consistency of natural/plain yogurt.

Put the romaine or cos lettuce in a large serving bowl. Lightly toss the avocado in lemon juice to stop it discolouring and add to the bowl with half the croutons. Arrange the halved eggs on top and drizzle enough of the dressing over to lightly coat everything. Break the bacon into long shards and arrange them over the salad with the remaining croutons.

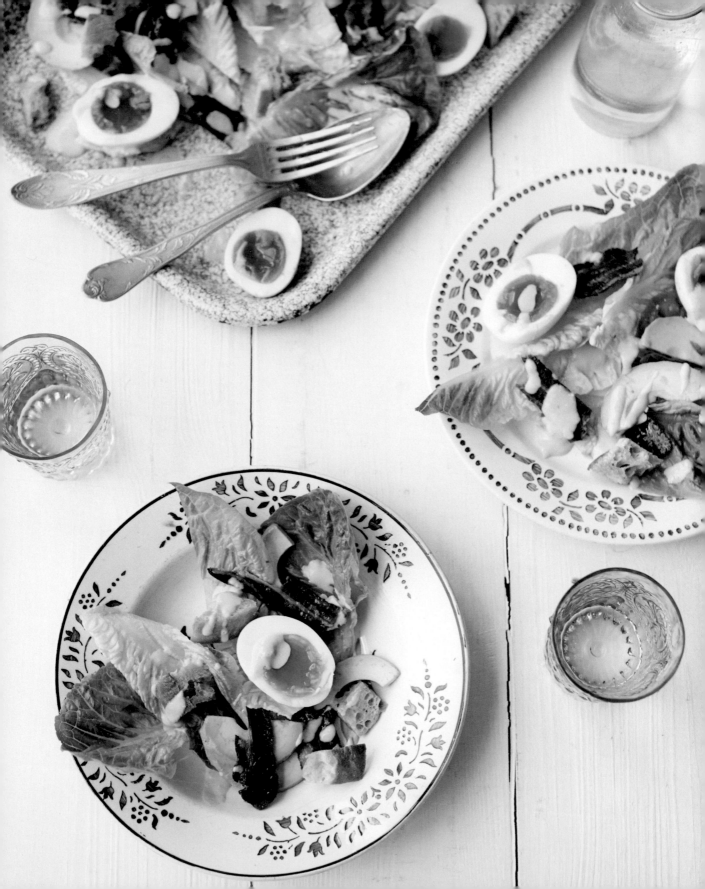

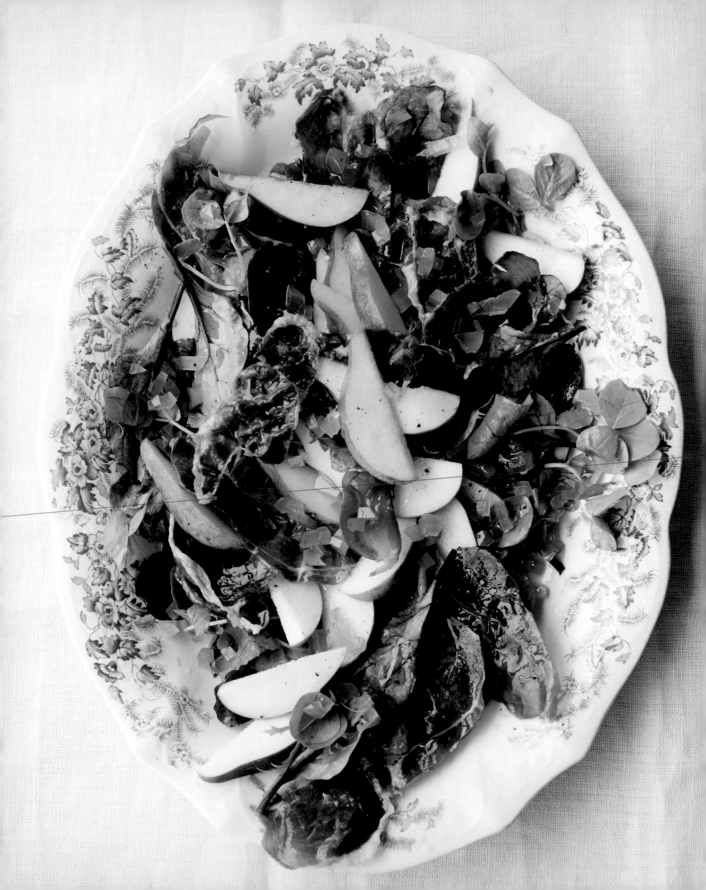

The combination of salty, crisp Italian air–dried ham with sweet, soft pear and a zing from the stem ginger makes this quite a sophisticated salad, perfect for a special occasion or appetizer.

Parma ham, pear & stem ginger salad

8 slices Parma ham
2 balls stem ginger, diced, plus 1 tablespoon syrup from the jar
125 g/4¼ oz. mixed baby leaf herb salad
50 g/⅓ cup pea shoots
2 pears, halved, cored and cut into long wedges

DRESSING
4 tablespoons extra virgin olive oil, preferably a fruity flavoured one
2 tablespoons freshly squeezed lemon juice
sea salt and freshly ground black pepper

Serves 4

Place the slices of Parma ham in a dry, non-stick frying pan/skillet and cook over a medium heat for 3–4 minutes, turning once, until just crisp. Remove from the pan, drain on paper towels, and lightly brush the top of each slice while still warm with the ginger syrup.

Meanwhile, mix together all the ingredients for the dressing and season with salt and pepper.

Put the salad leaves and pea shoots on a serving plate and top with the pears and stem ginger. Spoon as much of the dressing over as needed, then toss gently until lightly coated. Arrange the slices of Parma ham on top and serve immediately.

PEARS
For the best flavour, make sure the pears are at the peak of ripeness. You don't want them to be hard and flavourless, or so ripe that they turn to mush when sliced.

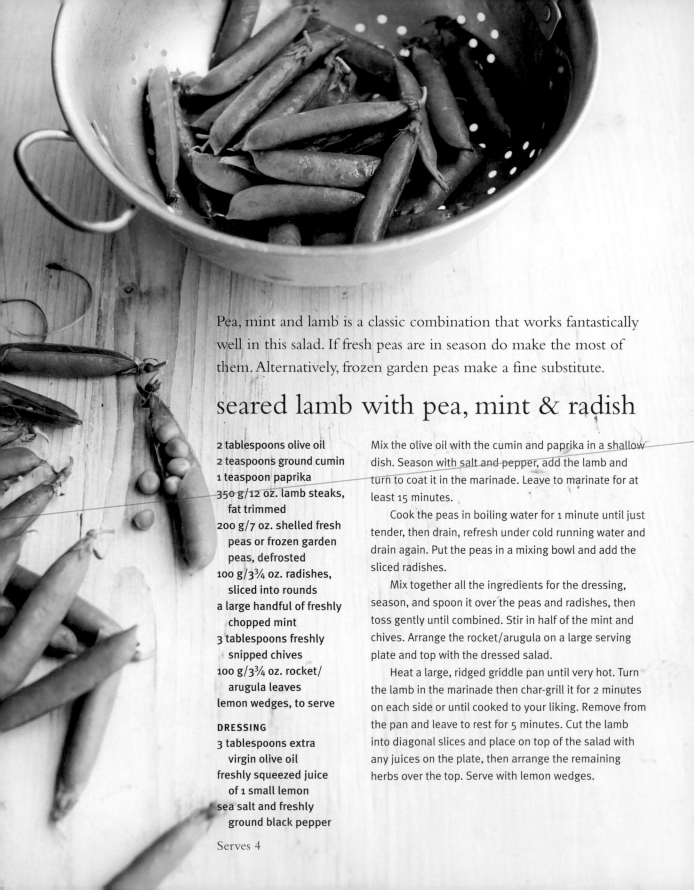

Pea, mint and lamb is a classic combination that works fantastically well in this salad. If fresh peas are in season do make the most of them. Alternatively, frozen garden peas make a fine substitute.

seared lamb with pea, mint & radish

2 tablespoons olive oil
2 teaspoons ground cumin
1 teaspoon paprika
350 g/12 oz. lamb steaks,
   fat trimmed
200 g/7 oz. shelled fresh
   peas or frozen garden
   peas, defrosted
100 g/3¾ oz. radishes,
   sliced into rounds
a large handful of freshly
   chopped mint
3 tablespoons freshly
   snipped chives
100 g/3¾ oz. rocket/
   arugula leaves
lemon wedges, to serve

DRESSING
3 tablespoons extra
   virgin olive oil
freshly squeezed juice
   of 1 small lemon
sea salt and freshly
   ground black pepper

Serves 4

Mix the olive oil with the cumin and paprika in a shallow dish. Season with salt and pepper, add the lamb and turn to coat it in the marinade. Leave to marinate for at least 15 minutes.

Cook the peas in boiling water for 1 minute until just tender, then drain, refresh under cold running water and drain again. Put the peas in a mixing bowl and add the sliced radishes.

Mix together all the ingredients for the dressing, season, and spoon it over the peas and radishes, then toss gently until combined. Stir in half of the mint and chives. Arrange the rocket/arugula on a large serving plate and top with the dressed salad.

Heat a large, ridged griddle pan until very hot. Turn the lamb in the marinade then char-grill it for 2 minutes on each side or until cooked to your liking. Remove from the pan and leave to rest for 5 minutes. Cut the lamb into diagonal slices and place on top of the salad with any juices on the plate, then arrange the remaining herbs over the top. Serve with lemon wedges.

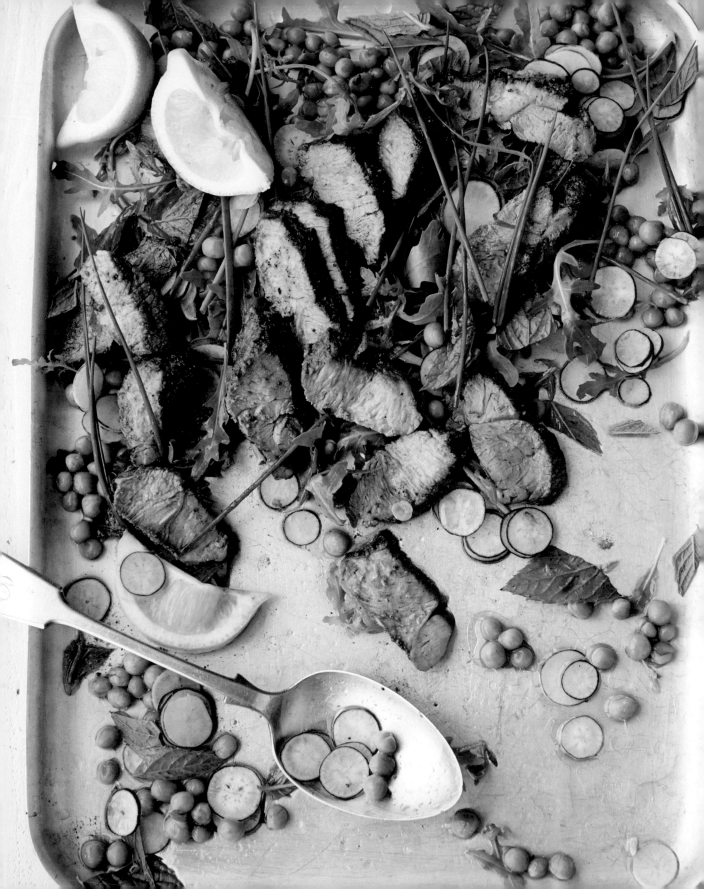

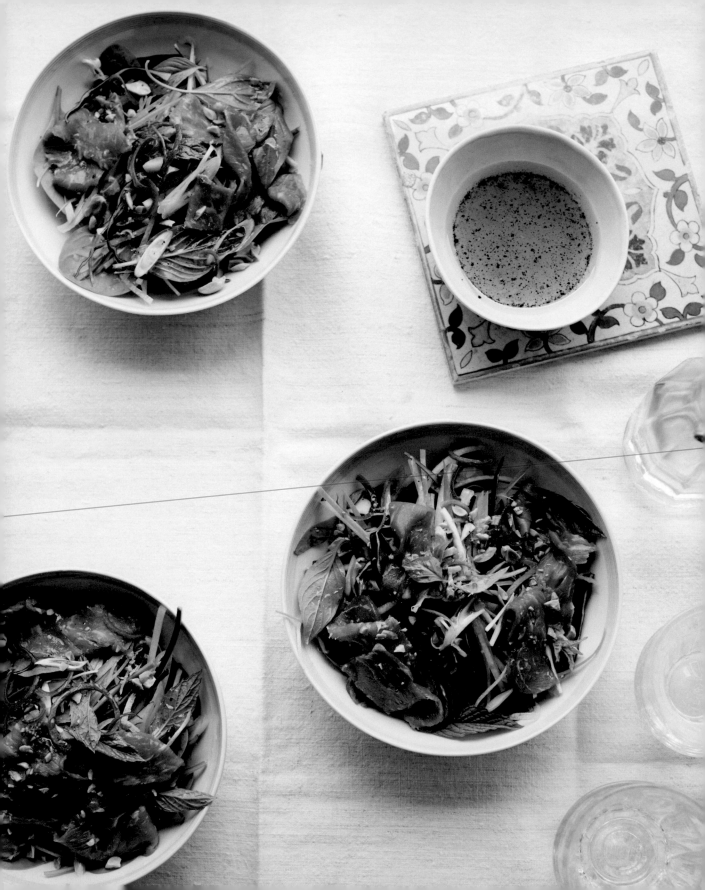

Fresh and fragrant, this salad is full of vibrant flavours with its sweet and sour dressing and lots of crisp vegetables. As a twist, the salad is topped with carpaccio of beef. To make the beef easier to cut into thin slices, freeze it first to firm up and use a very sharp, long-bladed knife. Choose a thick piece of beef, preferably a centre cut.

Vietnamese-style beef salad

200 g/7 oz. sirloin steak
2 handfuls of baby
    spinach leaves
1 carrot, sliced into
    thin strips
1 small cucumber,
    quartered lengthways,
    seeded and cut
    into thin strips
2 handfuls of finely
    shredded red cabbage
2 spring onions/
    scallions, thinly
    sliced diagonally
a handful of Thai basil
    leaves, roughly torn
a handful of mint leaves,
    roughly chopped
1 medium red chilli/
    chile, seeded and
    thinly sliced
30 g/¼ cup roasted
    unsalted peanuts,
    roughly chopped

VIETNAMESE DRESSING
3 tablespoons groundnut/
    peanut oil
2 tablespoons fish sauce
freshly squeezed juice
    of 1 lime
1 teaspoon caster/
    superfine sugar
sea salt and freshly
    ground black pepper

Serves 4

Put the steak in the freezer for 30 minutes to firm up and to make it easier to slice.

While the steak is in the freezer, mix together all the ingredients for the dressing and season to taste.

Divide the spinach between 4 serving plates and top with the carrot, cucumber and red cabbage. Spoon enough of the dressing over to coat and toss lightly until combined.

Remove the steak from the freezer and using a very sharp, long-bladed knife, cut into thin, elegant slices. Place the cut slices on a plate and cover with clingfilm/plastic wrap to prevent them discolouring; if you put clingfilm/plastic wrap between each layer of beef, you will be able to separate them easily.

Arrange the steak on top of the salad, season and sprinkle the spring onions/scallions, herbs, chilli/chile and peanuts over the top. Spoon more dressing over to taste, and serve immediately.

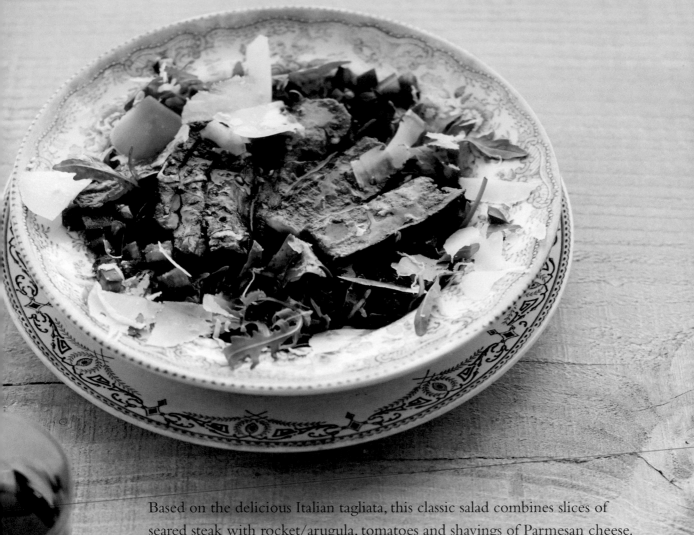

Based on the delicious Italian tagliata, this classic salad combines slices of seared steak with rocket/arugula, tomatoes and shavings of Parmesan cheese. Serve with roasted potato wedges or slices of ciabatta.

beef tagliata

2 thick beef steaks, about 250 g/9 oz. each, such as rib-eye or sirloin, at room temperature
1 tablespoon extra virgin olive oil, plus extra for drizzling
125 g/4¼ oz. rocket/ arugula leaves
4 vine-ripened tomatoes, seeded and diced

4 teaspoons balsamic vinegar
60 g/2 oz. Parmesan cheese, shaved into thin slices
sea salt and freshly ground black pepper

Serves 4

Brush the steaks with olive oil and season. Heat a large ridged griddle pan over a high heat. Sear the steaks for about 2–3 minutes on each side, turning once or twice. Leave to rest, covered with foil, for 5 minutes.

Meanwhile, make the salad. Arrange the rocket/ arugula and tomatoes over 4 serving plates.

Cut the steak into 1 cm/½ in. slices and arrange on top of the salad. Spoon any pan juices over and drizzle with the balsamic vinegar and extra olive oil. Sprinkle the Parmesan cheese shavings over and season with salt and pepper.

This is a sophisticated salad that could be served as an appetizer for a special occasion, or as a light meal with slices of walnut bread.

smoked venison, sour cherry & walnut salad

4 UK large/US extra-
  large eggs
150 g/5 oz. mixed red
  leaf salad
125 g/4¼ oz. artichoke
  hearts in oil, drained,
  halved or quartered
  if large
50 g/½ cup walnut
  halves, toasted
30 g/¼ cup dried sour
  cherries, halved if large
150 g/5 oz. cooked
  smoked venison, sliced

WALNUT DRESSING
4 tablespoons walnut oil
1 tablespoon extra virgin
  olive oil
2 tablespoons white
  wine vinegar
sea salt and freshly
  ground black pepper

Serves 4

Put the eggs in a small pan, cover generously with water and bring to the boil. Turn off the heat and leave for 3 minutes, until the white is set but the yolk remains runny. Cool the eggs slightly under cold running water, then peel.

Meanwhile, mix together the ingredients for the dressing and season with salt and pepper.

Arrange the salad leaves on 4 serving plates. Top with the artichoke hearts, walnuts and cherries. Spoon enough of the dressing over to lightly coat the salad. Toss gently, then top with the venison and halved, soft-boiled eggs.

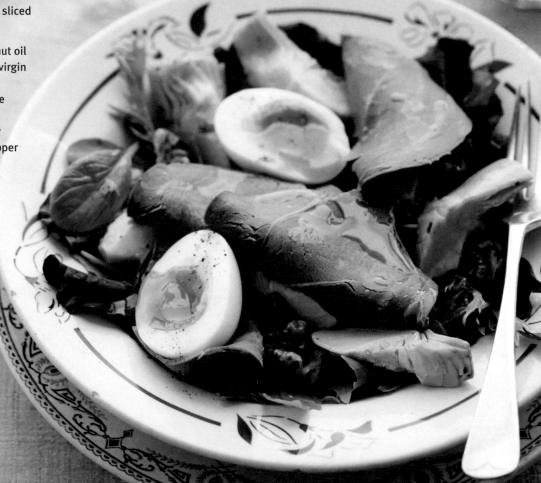

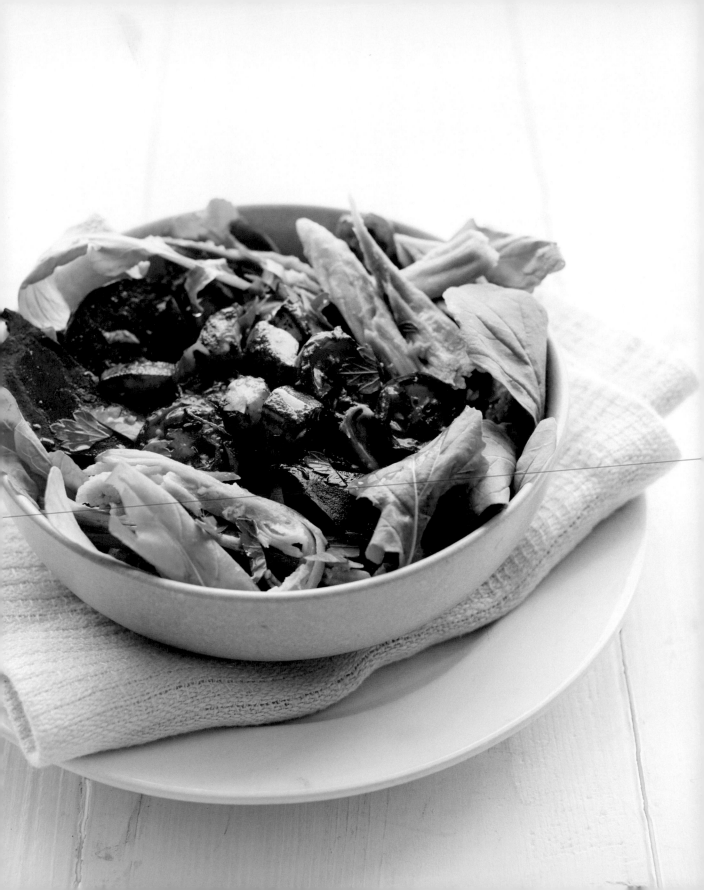

Salads don't have to be restricted to the warmer summer months; this winter alternative makes a simple meal served with crusty bread. It is equally good served at room temperature for lunch, and you could use cooked beetroot/beets and canned lentils for a quick meal.

warm ham hock, beetroot & lentil salad

3 uncooked beetroot/
    beets, washed and
    each one cut into
    8 wedges
4 tablespoons extra
    virgin olive oil
200 g/7 oz. dried green
    lentils
2 large garlic cloves,
    finely chopped
1 courgette/zucchini,
    quartered and diced
175 g/6 oz. vine-ripened
    cherry tomatoes,
    halved
2 tablespoons thyme
    leaves
2 heaped teaspoons
    Dijon mustard

freshly squeezed juice
    of 1 lemon
100 g/3¾ oz. rocket/
    arugula leaves
a handful of roughly
    chopped flat leaf
    parsley
180 g/6 oz. cooked
    smoked ham hock,
    shredded
sea salt and freshly
    ground black pepper

Serves 4

Preheat the oven to 200°C (400°F) Gas 6.

Put the beetroot/beets in a roasting pan and brush with 1 tablespoon of the olive oil. Season and bake in the preheated oven for 40–45 minutes, turning once, until tender.

Meanwhile, put the lentils in a pan and pour enough water over to cover. Bring to the boil, then turn the heat down, part-cover, and simmer for 20–25 minutes until tender, then drain.

Heat the remaining oil in a large sauté pan over a medium heat and fry the garlic, courgette/zucchini and tomatoes for 3 minutes until softened. Stir in the thyme, mustard and lemon juice until combined.

Remove from the heat and fold in the rocket/ arugula, parsley, ham hock and lentils, taking care not to break up the lentils, and allow the heat of the pan to wilt the leaves. Season before folding in the roasted beetroot/beets, then serve while still warm or let cool to room temperature.

HAM HOCK

For convenience this salad uses cooked ham hock, which is now readily available. If time allows though, it's far more economical to cook your own; not only will you have a sufficient amount of ham for other dishes, you'll also have a flavoursome stock.

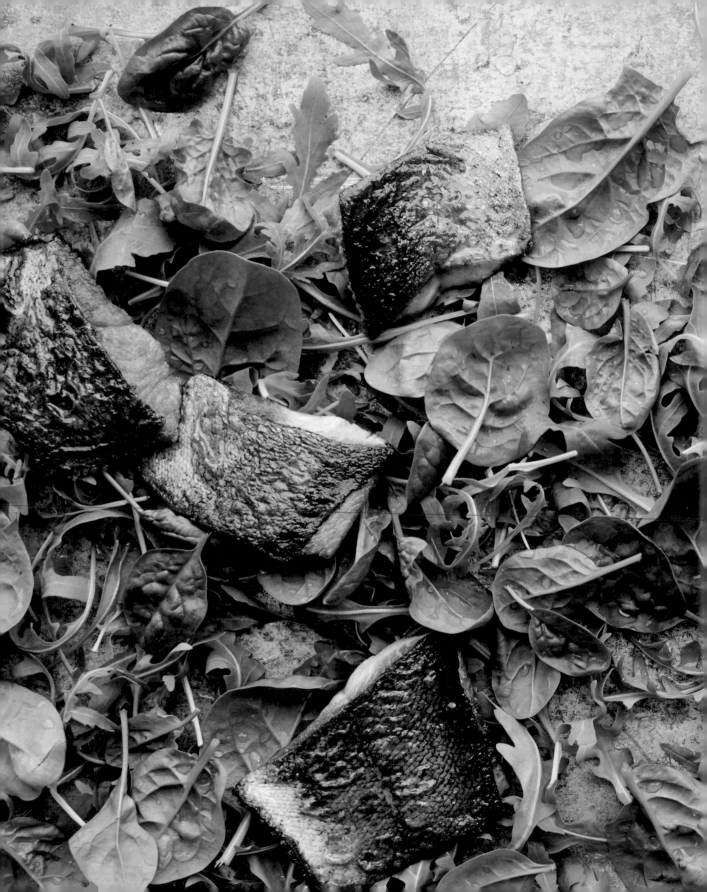

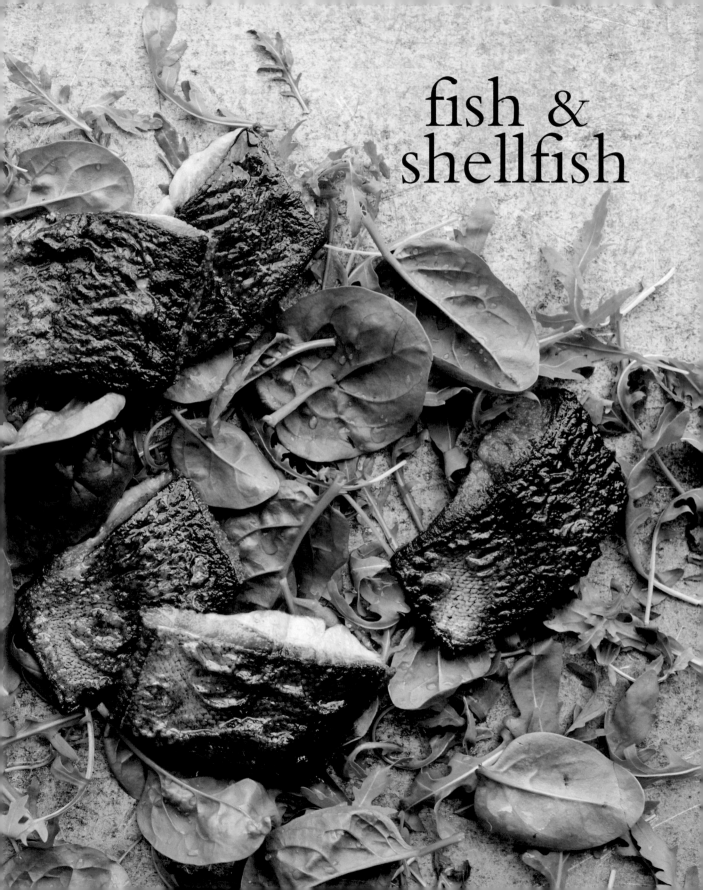

fish &
shellfish

This salad has a Scandinavian feel and is full of fresh, vibrant flavours, topped off with a creamy dill dressing. Serve with slices of rye bread or new potatoes.

Use the freshest fish possible for this gravadlax. Ideally, buy a mid-cut fillet, which will be just the right thickness to take on the flavours.

smoked salmon, quail's egg & radish salad

10 quail's eggs
1 round/butterhead lettuce, leaves torn
100 g/3¾ oz. radishes, sliced
2 cooked beetroot/beets in natural juice, diced
1 banana shallot, diced
1–2 tablespoons cold-pressed rapeseed oil, for drizzling
160 g/5½ oz. smoked salmon, torn into pieces
a handful of chives, snipped
a few alfalfa sprouts

CREAMY DILL DRESSING
4 tablespoons mayonnaise (see page 12)
4 tablespoons crème fraîche
freshly squeezed juice of 1 small lemon
2 tablespoons roughly chopped dill
sea salt and freshly ground black pepper

Serves 4

Cook the quail's eggs in a pan of boiling water for 2 minutes, drain and cool under cold running water, then peel and halve.

Arrange the lettuce leaves on 4 serving plates and top with the radishes, beetroot/beets and shallot. Drizzle over the rapeseed oil.

Mix together all the ingredients for the dill dressing and season with salt and pepper.

Top the salad with the smoked salmon, quail's eggs, chives and alfalfa, then add a good spoonful of the creamy dill dressing.

home-cured salmon with gin & beetroot

500 g/1 lb 2 oz. wild salmon fillet, pin-boned
3 uncooked beetroot/ beets, coarsely grated
80 g/3 oz. rock salt
80 g/3 oz. white sugar
finely grated zest of 2 lemons
2 handfuls of snipped dill
2 tablespoons gin

HERBY MAYONNAISE
6 tablespoons mayonnaise (see page 12)
1 tablespoon chopped drained capers

2 tablespoons freshly snipped chives
2 tablespoons freshly snipped dill
freshly squeezed juice of ½ lemon
¼ red onion, diced

TO SERVE
beetroot and watercress salad
slices of brown bread, buttered if you like
lemon wedges

Serves 4–6

Lay the fish, skin-side up, on a sheet of baking parchment. Mix the beetroot/beets, salt and sugar together and spread half the mixture over the skin. Turn the fish over and spread the remaining beetroot/beet mixture over the flesh, making sure it is completely covered. Wrap the fish in the parchment, then wrap tightly in two layers of clingfilm/plastic wrap. Place in a non-metallic dish, cover with clingfilm/plastic wrap and put it in the refrigerator for 24 hours, turning the fish after 12 hours.

Unwrap the fish and brush off the marinade. Rinse the salmon under cold running water, then pat dry with paper towels and return to the dish, skin-side down. Mix the lemon zest, dill and gin together and spread the mixture over the salmon, pressing it into the flesh. Cover with clingfilm/plastic wrap and chill for 24 hours.

To serve, mix together the mayonnaise ingredients and slice the salmon thinly at an angle.

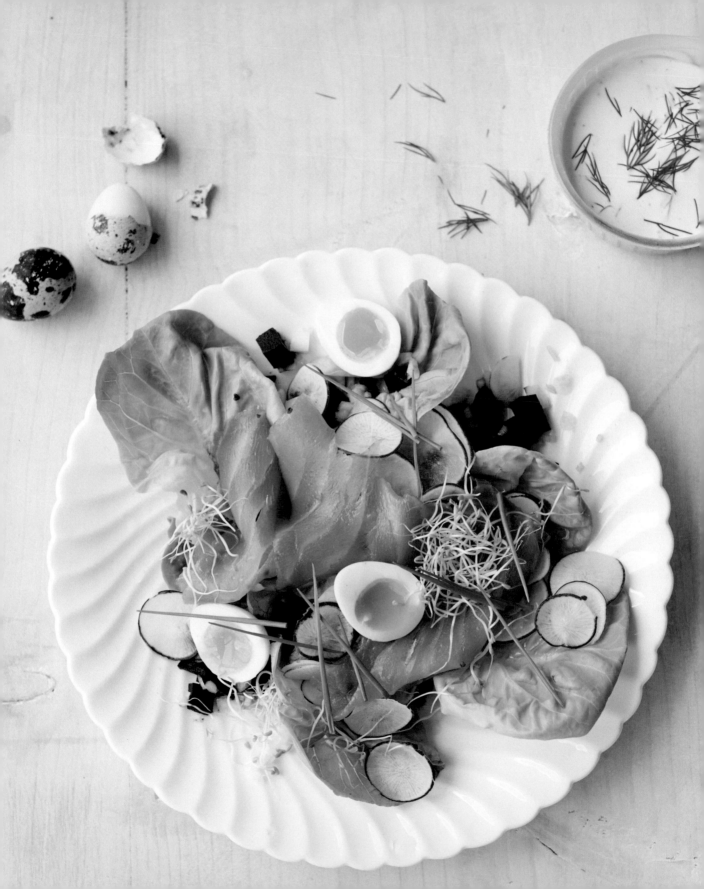

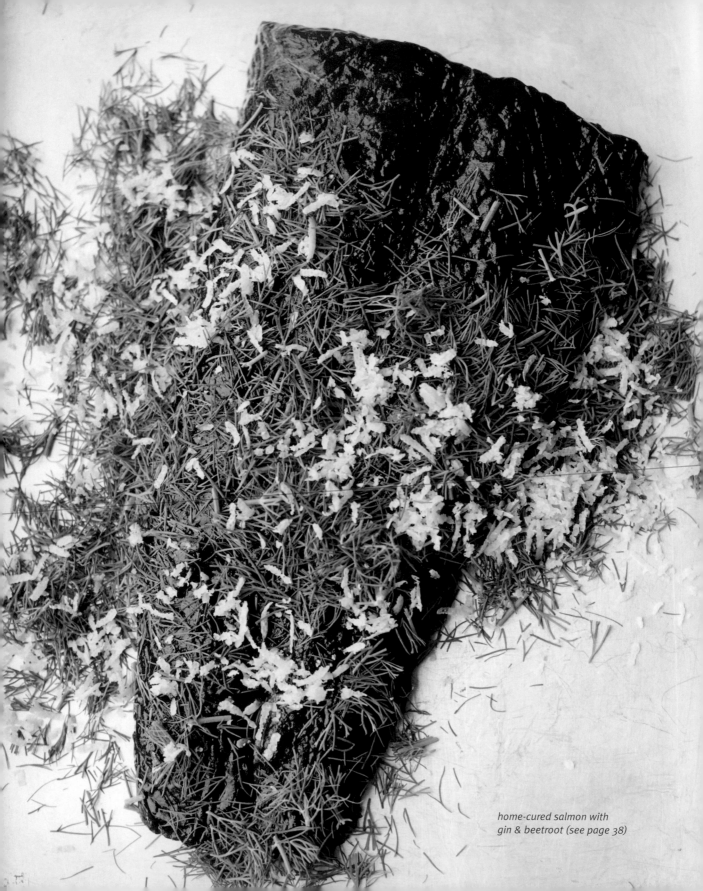

home-cured salmon with
gin & beetroot (see page 38)

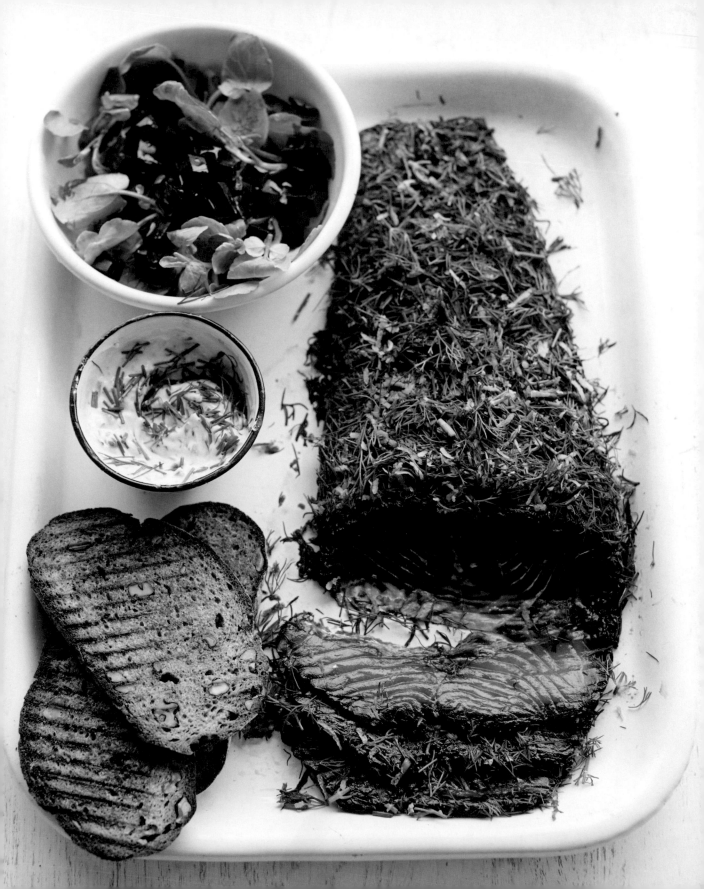

Black rice not only looks impressive, especially when combined with the pink-fleshed salmon and vibrant orange of mango as in this salad, it also has a great nutty flavour and holds its shape when cooked.

Asian salmon, black rice & mango salad

300 g/11 oz. black rice,
   rinsed
4 wild salmon fillets
sesame oil, for brushing
1 small red onion,
   thinly sliced
10-cm/4-in. piece
   cucumber, thinly sliced
   into ribbons
1 mango, peeled, stoned/
   pitted and sliced
a handful of mint leaves
60 g/2 oz. pea shoots
1 tablespoon toasted
   sesame seeds
sea salt and freshly
   ground black pepper

DRESSING
3 tablespoons light
   soy sauce
2 tablespoons mirin
1 heaped teaspoon
   caster/superfine sugar
1-cm/½-in. piece fresh
   root ginger, peeled and
   finely diced

Serves 4

Put the rice in a pan and cover generously with cold water. Bring to the boil, then turn the heat down to low, cover, and simmer for 25 minutes or until tender. Drain and transfer the rice to a large bowl.

Meanwhile, preheat the grill/broiler to high and line a grill/broiling pan with foil. Brush the salmon with sesame oil, season, then place, skin-side down, in the grill/broiling pan. Grill/broil for 5 minutes on each side or until the skin is crisp and golden and the salmon is just cooked. Remove from the grill/broiler, peel away the skin, cut into strips and reserve.

Mix together all the ingredients for the dressing and season with black pepper.

Add the onion, cucumber, mango and mint to the bowl with the rice, pour enough of the dressing over to coat and lightly toss until combined.

Put the pea shoots on four serving plates and top with the rice mixture. Place the salmon on top or flake it and stir it into the rice, sprinkle over the sesame seeds and arrange some of the crispy salmon skin on top before serving.

SALMON
There is much debate surrounding wild and farmed salmon, but it is universally agreed that both are good sources of beneficial omega-3 fatty acids. Getting the cooking time right is crucial for the best flavour, as salmon can soon become dry – it should retain a strand of deeper pink flesh running through the centre.

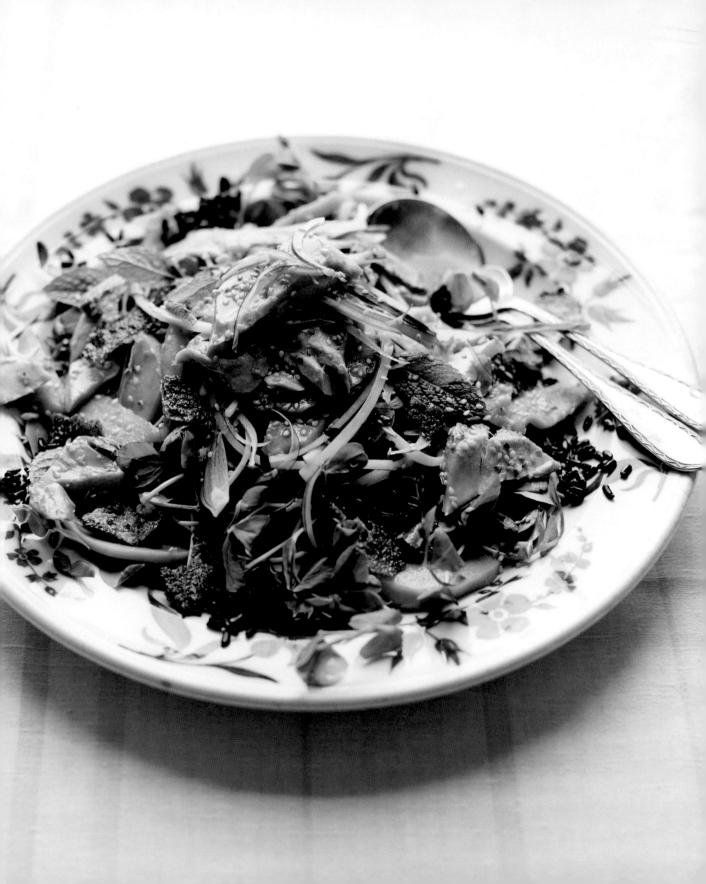

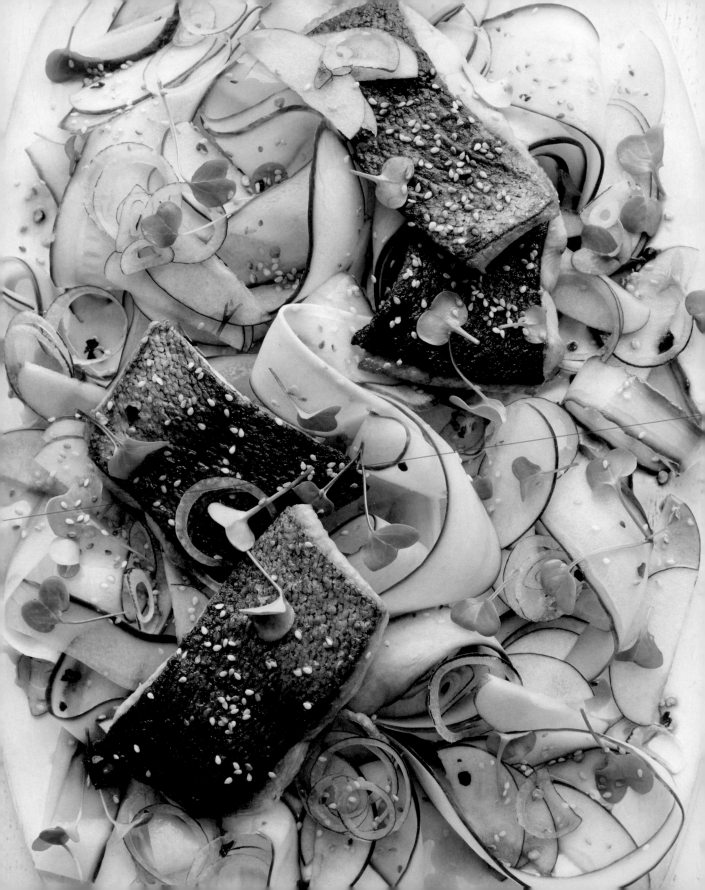

This pretty Peruvian-style salad has a typically fusion-style dressing, featuring the citrus tang of fresh orange and lime combined with Japanese mirin and tamari.

pink trout, cucumber & apple salad

4 pink trout fillets, about 560 g/1¼ lb total weight, rinsed and patted dry
sesame oil, for brushing
1 small cucumber
2 red-skinned apples, quartered, cored and thinly sliced
1 small red onion, thinly sliced into rings
2 teaspoons toasted sesame seeds
a handful of broccoli sprouts or micro herbs
sea salt and freshly ground black pepper

CITRUS & MIRIN DRESSING
freshly squeezed juice of ½ orange
freshly squeezed juice of 1 lime, plus extra for the apples
2 tablespoons mirin
½ teaspoon dried chilli/ hot pepper flakes
3–4 tablespoons tamari or light soy sauce, to taste

Serves 4

Preheat the grill/broiler to medium-high and line the grill/broiling pan with foil. Brush the trout with sesame oil and season.

While the grill/broiler is heating, mix together all the ingredients for the dressing, adding the tamari to taste.

Using a vegetable peeler, slice the cucumber into ribbons, discarding the seeds when you reach the centre. Arrange the cucumber on 4 serving plates. Toss the apples in a little lime juice to prevent them discolouring and arrange on top of the cucumber.

Grill/broil the trout, skin-side down first, for 6 minutes, then turn it over and grill/broil for another 4–6 minutes until cooked, depending on the thickness of the fillets. Peel off and discard the skin, if you like, and leave the trout to cool slightly before placing on top of the apples. Top with the red onion, then spoon the dressing over. Finish with a sprinkling of sesame seeds and broccoli sprouts.

MICRO HERBS

These small plant seedlings can be combined with other salad leaves to add both taste and texture, or simply sprinkled over the top of a salad as a final flourish. For their size, they pack a powerful punch – look for rocket/arugula, coriander/ cilantro, basil and parsley, or micro greens such as broccoli, spinach, fennel or mizuna.

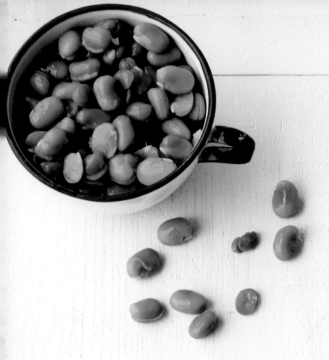

This vibrant salad has a Nordic feel and makes a perfect light lunch, served with rye bread. You can find pickled herrings at deli counters or they are sold in jars; they make a quick, nutritious and convenient addition to a meal.

herring, broad bean & beetroot salad with horseradish dressing

200 g/7 oz. shelled
  broad/fava beans
2 Ruby Gem/Bibb
  lettuces, leaves sliced
1 red chicory/Belgian
  endive, leaves
  separated and sliced
2 raw beetroot/beets,
  peeled and grated
1 small red onion, diced
250 g/9 oz. pickled
  herrings in dill, drained
a handful of alfalfa and
  radish sprouts
2 hard-boiled eggs,
  yolks only
rye bread, to serve
  (optional)

HORSERADISH DRESSING
3 tablespoons olive oil
1½ tablespoons cider
  vinegar
2 tablespoons creamed
  horseradish
2 tablespoons single/
  light cream
sea salt and freshly
  ground black pepper

Serves 4

Steam the broad/fava beans for 2–3 minutes until tender, then refresh under cold running water. Peel off the grey outer shells to reveal the green beans.

Meanwhile, for the dressing, whisk together the oil and vinegar. Add the horseradish and cream, and whisk again until combined. Season and set aside.

Arrange the lettuce and chicory/Belgian endive on 4 serving plates, then top with the beetroot/beets, red onion and cooked broad/fava beans. Drizzle over three-quarters of the dressing and toss gently until combined. Top with the herrings and sprouts and grate the egg yolks over, then drizzle with the remaining dressing.

Serve on rye bread, if you like.

BROAD/FAVA BEANS
These can be eaten with their greeny-grey shell, but broad/fava beans taste sweeter and look prettier if the shell is removed to reveal the bright green bean inside. If fresh beans are unavailable, you can use frozen instead.

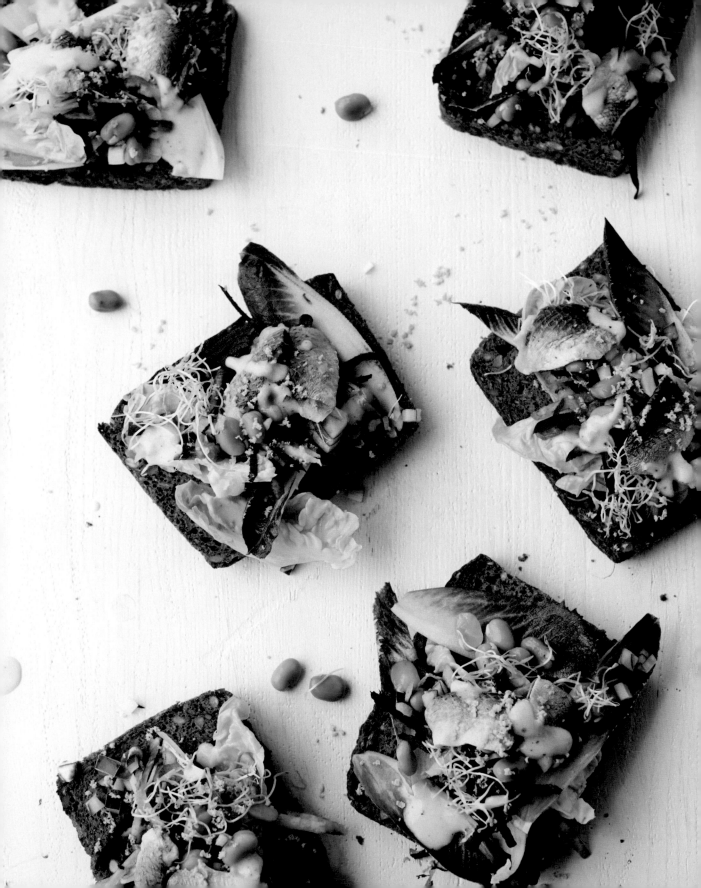

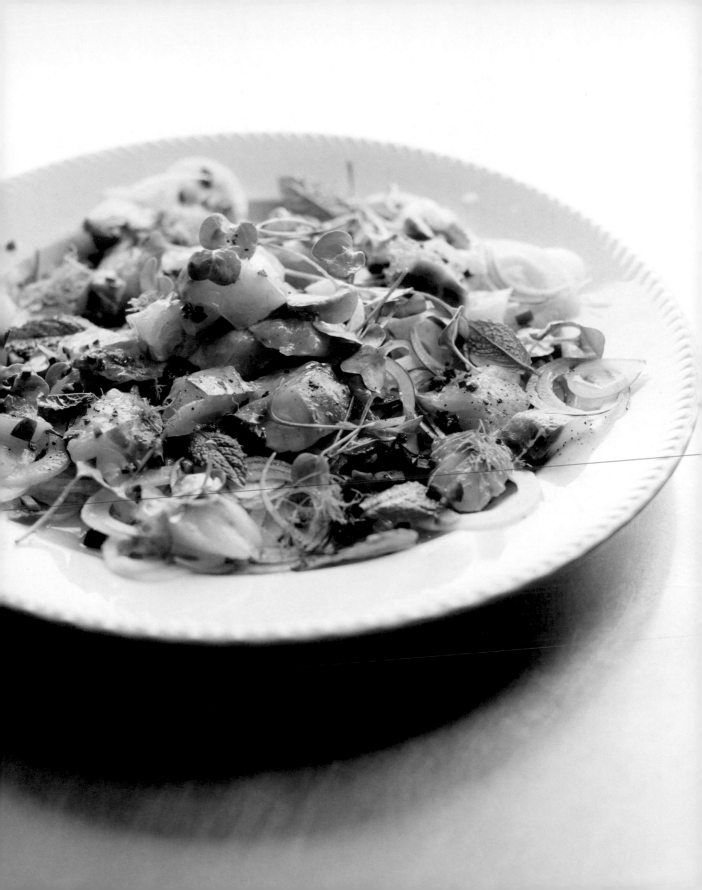

Ceviche, a Peruvian way of semi-poaching fish in citrus juice, looks impressive but is actually very simple to make. Fresh, light and vibrant, the secret to the success of this dish is to use ultra-fresh fish.

sea bass ceviche with fennel

400 g/14 oz. sea bass
  fillets, skin and bones
  removed, cut into
  2-cm/¾-in. squares
1 large fennel bulb,
  halved crossways and
  cut into thin strips,
  fronds reserved
1 small red onion, halved
  and thinly sliced
1 red pepper/bell pepper,
  seeded and finely
  chopped
leaves from 2 long sprigs
  of mint
a handful of mixed radish
  and broccoli sprouts
extra virgin olive oil,
  for drizzling

DRESSING
freshly squeezed juice
  of 3 limes
freshly squeezed juice
  of 1 orange
1 medium-sized red
  chilli/chile, seeded
  and diced
sea salt and freshly
  ground black pepper

Serves 4

Mix together all the ingredients for the dressing in a bowl, season generously with salt, cover and chill for 30 minutes.

Assemble the ceviche shortly before serving. Put the sea bass in a bowl, pour the dressing over and turn until combined. Leave to stand for 3 minutes while you prepare the salad; you don't want to "cook" the fish in the juice so be mindful of the time.

Arrange the fennel, onion, red pepper/bell pepper and mint leaves on four plates. Top with the sea bass and spoon some of the dressing over each serving, turn gently until combined, then sprinkle with the sprouts and fennel fronds. Drizzle over a little olive oil, season with black pepper and serve.

RADISH AND BROCCOLI SPROUTS
Loaded with vitamins and minerals, sprouted radish and broccoli seeds have a distinctive peppery, spicy taste.
To have a go at sprouting your own, see page 8.

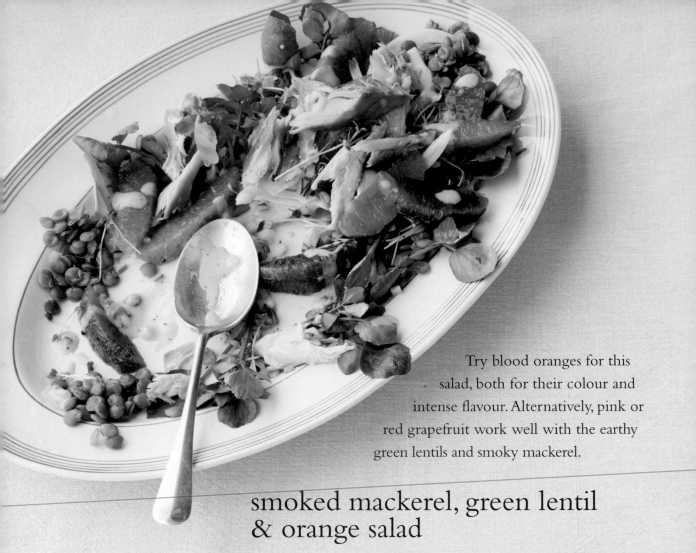

Try blood oranges for this salad, both for their colour and intense flavour. Alternatively, pink or red grapefruit work well with the earthy green lentils and smoky mackerel.

smoked mackerel, green lentil & orange salad

200 g/7 oz. dried green lentils

125 g/4¼ oz. watercress, thick stems removed, leaves torn into sprigs

2 handfuls of salad cress/fine curled cress

1 small red onion, diced

1 fennel bulb, cut into long, thin slices

4 large smoked mackerel fillets, skin and any bones removed

2 blood oranges, peeled, pith removed and segmented

DRESSING

4 tablespoons cold-pressed rapeseed oil or olive oil

2 tablespoons apple cider vinegar

5 teaspoons tartare sauce

2 tablespoons crème fraîche

sea salt and freshly ground black pepper

Serves 4

Put the lentils in a pan and cover with water. Bring to the boil, then turn the heat down, part-cover, and simmer for 20–25 minutes until tender. Drain and transfer to a large, shallow salad bowl.

Meanwhile, mix together the oil and vinegar for the dressing until combined, then whisk in the tartare sauce and crème fraîche, and season. Add a little water, if needed, to make a pouring consistency.

Add the watercress, salad cress/fine curled cress, onion and fennel to the lentils, spoon over half the dressing and toss until combined.

Flake the mackerel into large, bite-sized pieces and arrange on top of the salad with the orange segments, then drizzle with the remaining dressing.

Canned fish, including sardines, mackerel and herrings, makes a useful and nutritious storecupboard standby. Adjust the amount of lime juice used in the dressing, depending on preference.

sardine, avocado & red onion salad

150 g/5 oz. soft mixed
   salad leaves, such as
   watercress, rocket/
   arugula and baby
   spinach
1 small red onion, halved
   and thinly sliced
2 avocados, peeled,
   halved, stoned/pitted
   and sliced
100 g/3¾ oz. mixed
   radishes, sliced
3 tablespoons freshly
   snipped chives
2 x 135-g/4½-oz. cans
   sardines in olive oil,
   drained, central spine
   removed
a large pinch of dried
   chilli/hot pepper
   flakes (optional)

DRESSING
3 tablespoons extra
   virgin olive oil
freshly squeezed juice
   of 1–2 limes, to taste
sea salt and freshly
   ground black pepper

Serves 4

First mix together all the ingredients for the dressing, season and taste, adding extra lime juice, if needed. Set aside.

Arrange the salad leaves, onion, avocados, radishes and half the chives on a large serving plate. Spoon half the dressing over and toss gently to combine. Top the salad with the sardines, extra dressing and the remaining chives and chilli/hot pepper flakes, if using, then serve.

Avocados make a deliciously creamy dressing when blended with tangy lime, fresh coriander/cilantro and fromage frais. If it seems a little thick for spooning over the prawns, loosen with a spoonful or two of water. If fresh peas are out of season, use cooked frozen garden peas that have been refreshed in water.

chilli prawns with avocado dressing

4 handfuls of torn red Little Gem/Bibb lettuce
1 red pepper/bell pepper, seeded and thinly sliced
50 g/2 oz. sugar snap peas, sliced diagonally
3 spring onions/ scallions, thinly sliced diagonally
100 g/3¾ oz. shelled fresh uncooked peas
350 g/12 oz. shelled cooked king prawns/ jumbo shrimp
1 red chilli/chile, seeded and finely sliced

AVOCADO DRESSING
2 avocados, peeled, halved, stoned/pitted and chopped
freshly squeezed juice of 2 limes
finely grated zest of 1 lime
6 tablespoons fromage frais or ricotta cheese
2 tablespoons freshly chopped coriander/ cilantro leaves, plus extra to serve
½ teaspoon dried chilli/ hot pepper flakes
sea salt and freshly ground black pepper

Serves 4

To make the avocado dressing, put all the ingredients in a blender and blend until smooth and creamy. Add a little water to loosen, if needed, and season well.

Arrange the lettuce leaves on a large serving plate, top with the red pepper/bell pepper, sugar snap peas, spring onions/scallions, peas and king prawns/jumbo shrimp. Spoon the avocado dressing on top before sprinkling with the sliced chilli/chile and extra coriander/cilantro, if you like.

AVOCADO
The knobbly, dark-skinned Hass avocado is considered the best variety. and its creamy, buttery flesh is full of beneficial oils and vitamins. To speed up ripening, put an avocado in a brown paper bag with a banana and wait for a day or so.

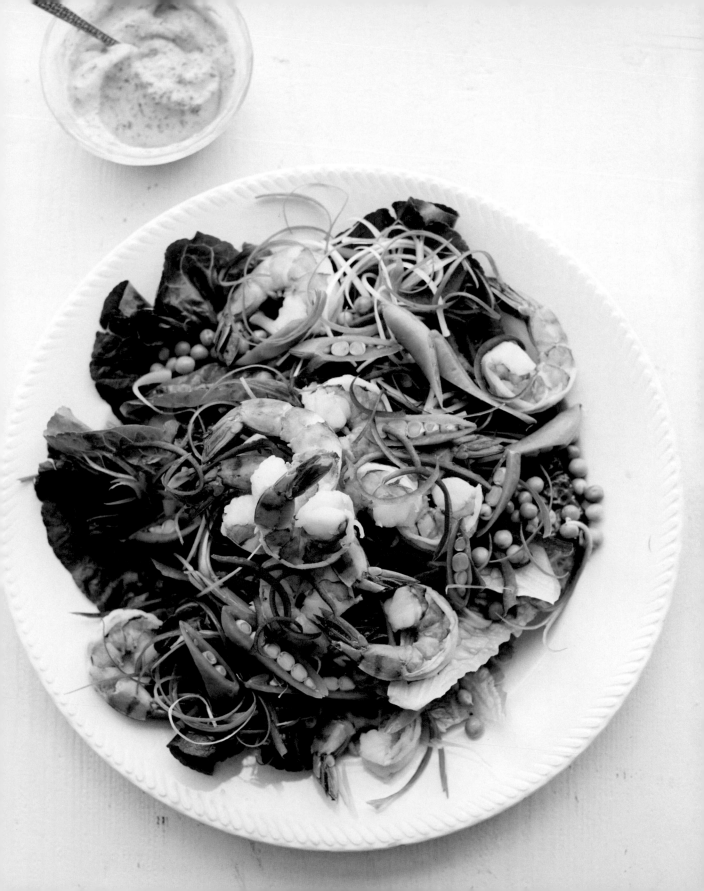

scallop & green papaya salad with lemongrass dressing

1 green papaya, peeled,
  halved and seeded
10-cm/4-in. piece
  cucumber
1 red chilli/chile, seeded
  and finely chopped
12 shelled prepared
  scallops
olive oil, for brushing
a handful of coriander/
  cilantro leaves
sea salt and freshly
  ground black pepper

LEMONGRASS DRESSING
freshly squeezed juice
  of 2 limes
1 tablespoon light brown
  soft sugar
1 tablespoon Thai fish
  sauce
2 teaspoons finely
  chopped peeled fresh
  root ginger
2 lemongrass stalks,
  outer leaves discarded
  and finely chopped
2 kaffir lime leaves, finely
  sliced

Serves 4

Shred the papaya using a mandoline or cut into long, thin strips. Slice the cucumber into ribbons using the mandoline or vegetable peeler, discarding the column of seeds in the centre. Put the papaya, cucumber and chilli/chile in a bowl.

Mix together all the ingredients for the dressing until the sugar dissolves, then pour it over the salad, toss until combined and leave for 15 minutes to allow the flavours to develop. Divide the salad between 4 serving plates.

Brush the scallops with a little oil and season. Heat a ridged griddle pan over a high heat and griddle the scallops for 1 minute on each side until just cooked. Arrange the scallops on top of the papaya salad and garnish with the coriander/cilantro leaves.

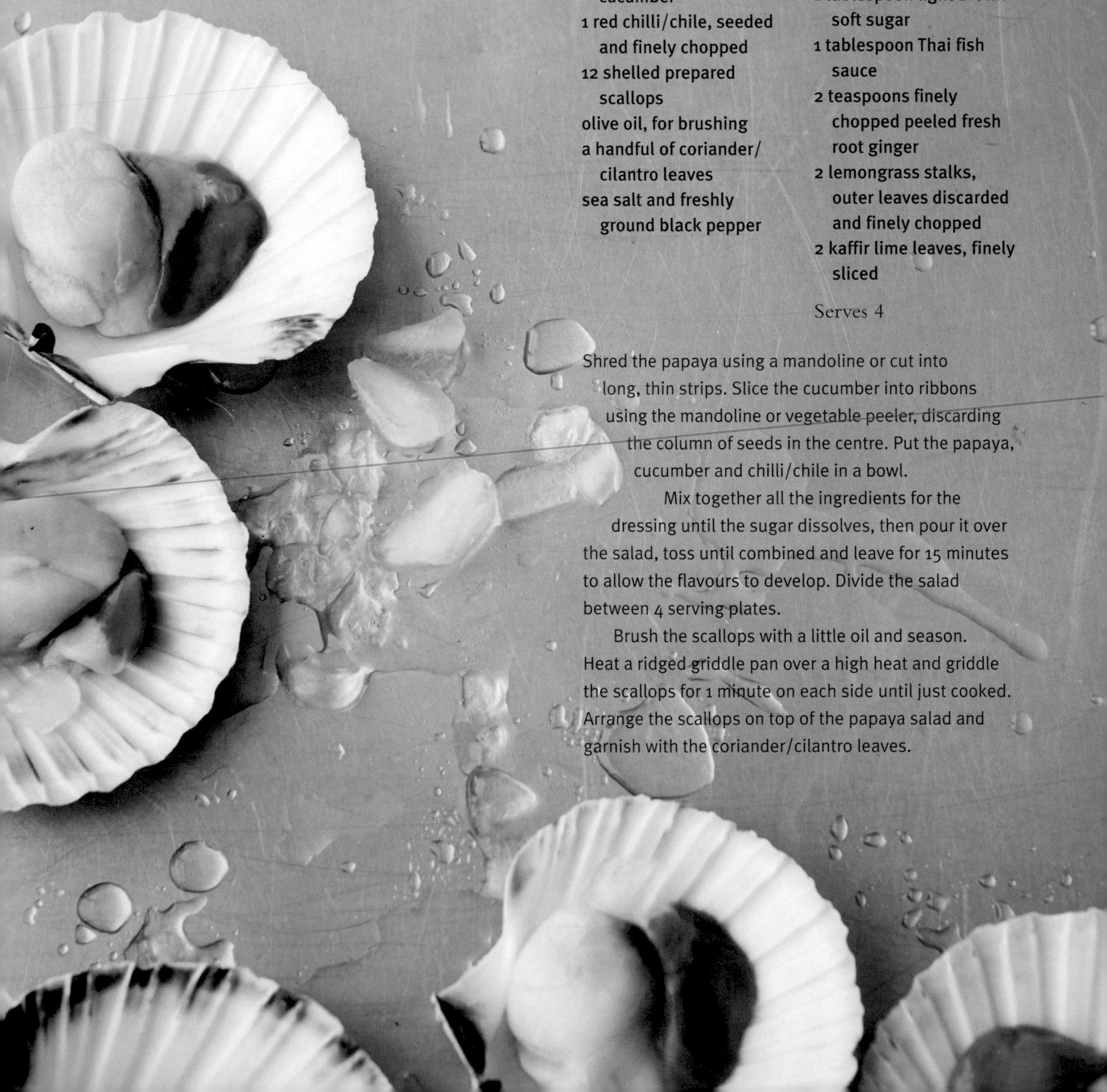

Inspired by the flavours of Thailand, this light and zingy salad is topped with seared scallops, but it would work equally well with other types of seafood such as salmon, sea bass, crab, king prawns/jumbo shrimp or squid. If you can't find green papaya, you could use green-fleshed melon.

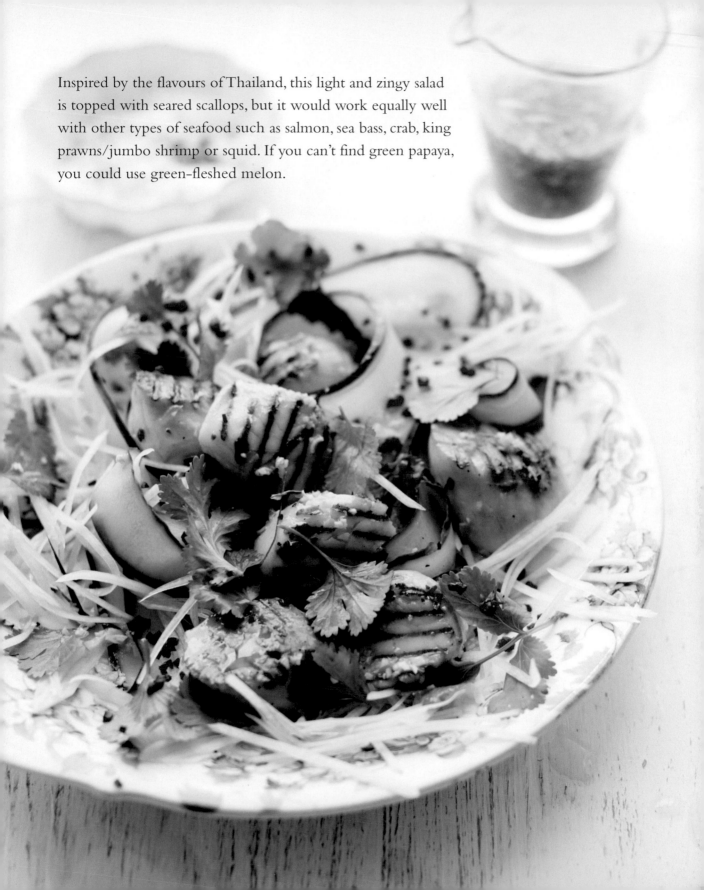

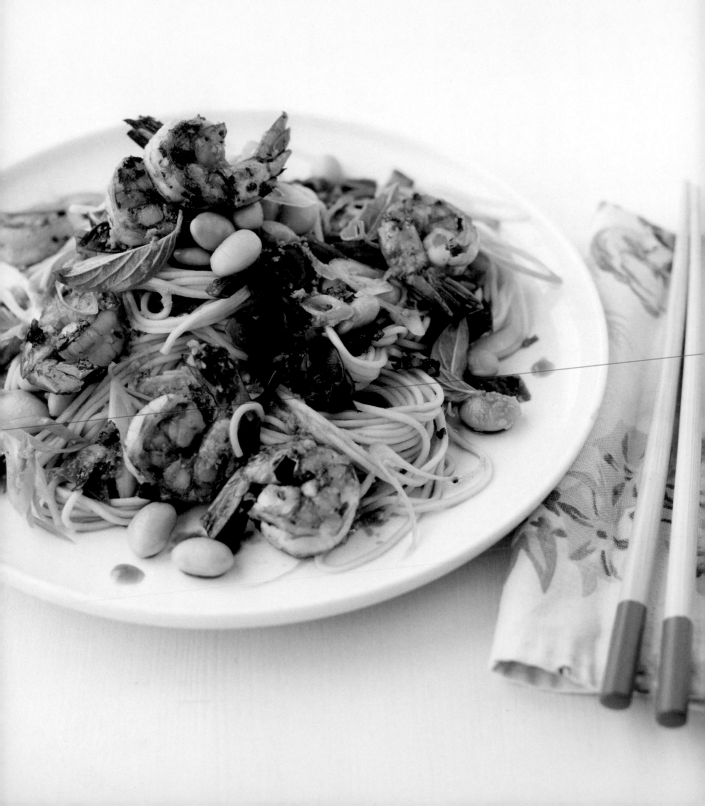

This main-meal salad calls for basil mint, a herb hybrid that combines two of our most popular varieties, yet Thai basil or a combination of basil and mint would work equally well if unavailable. This salad makes a perfect picnic lunch as it copes well with being transported.

prawn noodle salad with ginger-soy dressing

200 g/7 oz. shelled broad/fava beans
1 garlic clove, crushed
½ teaspoon dried chilli/hot pepper flakes
350 g/12 oz. raw peeled king prawns/jumbo shrimp
250 g/9 oz. fine egg noodles
12 g/¼ oz. dried wakame
3 spring onions/scallions, thinly sliced diagonally
a handful of basil mint leaves, chopped
1 tablespoon sunflower oil
sea salt

GINGER-SOY DRESSING
5 tablespoons light soy sauce
2 tablespoons sesame oil, plus 1 teaspoon
freshly squeezed juice of 1 lime
2.5-cm/1-in. piece fresh root ginger, peeled and finely grated

Serves 4

Steam the broad/fava beans for 2–3 minutes until tender, then refresh under cold running water. Pop the beans out of their grey outer shell to reveal a bright green bean.

Meanwhile, mix together the garlic, dried chilli/hot pepper flakes, 1 teaspoon of the sesame oil and a large pinch of salt in a shallow dish. Add the king prawns/jumbo shrimp and turn to coat them in the marinade.

Cook the noodles as instructed on the packet, then drain and refresh under cold running water. Put the wakame in a bowl, cover with cold water and leave for 3 minutes until rehydrated, then drain.

Put the noodles, broad/fava beans, wakame, spring onions/scallions and half the basil mint in a serving bowl. Mix together all the ingredients for the dressing, pour it over the noodle salad and toss until combined.

Heat the oil in a large frying pan/skillet over a medium heat and fry the king prawns/jumbo shrimp for 3 minutes, turning once, until pink and cooked through. Leave to cool slightly, then serve on top of the noodles, sprinkled with the remaining basil mint.

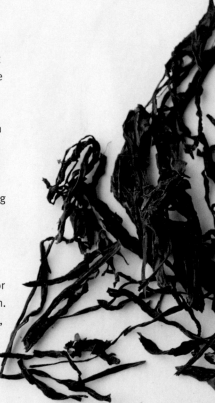

WAKAME
Look out for packs of dried wakame seaweed in health shops and large supermarkets. Popular in Japanese dishes, wakame is a good source of many minerals and takes mere minutes to rehydrate. It's a popular addition to miso soup.

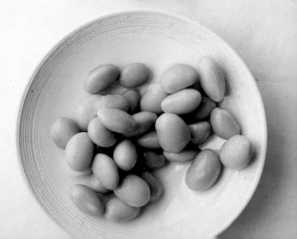

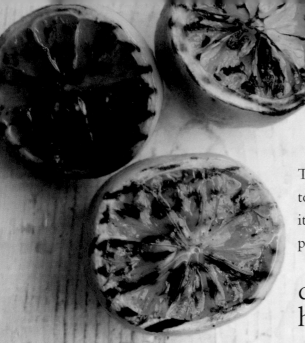

The beauty of squid is that it takes next to no time to cook – a minute or so is enough, any longer and it becomes tough and rubbery. Mizuna has a slightly peppery flavour, similar to rocket/arugula.

char-grilled squid with herb dressing

60 g/2 oz. mizuna or
  rocket/arugula leaves
100 g/3¾ oz. baby
  spinach leaves
4 vine-ripened tomatoes,
  quartered, seeded
  and diced
500 g/1 lb 2 oz. prepared
  and cleaned small squid
2 lemons, halved
2 tablespoons freshly
  snipped chives
1 red chilli/chile, seeded
  and cut into thin strips

HERB DRESSING
5 tablespoons extra
  virgin olive oil, plus
  extra for cooking
1 large garlic clove,
  crushed
2 handfuls of basil leaves
a handful of oregano
  leaves
freshly squeezed juice
  of ½ lemon
sea salt and freshly
  ground black pepper

Serves 4

To make the dressing, put all the ingredients in a mini-processor or blender and blend until the herbs are finely chopped. (You could also chop the herbs by hand.) Season the dressing and set aside.

Place the salad leaves on a large serving plate and arrange the tomatoes over the top.

Slice off the squid tentacles, if there are any. Open out the body of each squid and cut in half, then score the skin using the tip of a sharp knife into a diamond pattern. Into a large bowl, pour enough oil to coat the squid lightly and season. Add the squid (including the tentacles) and turn until coated in the oil.

Heat a large, ridged griddle pan over a medium-high heat and sear the lemon halves, cut-side down, pressing them down until caramelized in places. Remove from the griddle and set aside. Next, griddle the squid bodies in batches for 1½ minutes, turning once and pressing them down with a spatula, until cooked and charred in places. Griddle any tentacles, too, for 1 minute, turning once.

Arrange the squid on top of the salad, spoon the herb dressing over the top and garnish with the chives and chilli. Serve the char-grilled lemons on the side for squeezing over.

LEMON
To preserve their freshness most lemons are routinely waxed, but if you intend to use the zest in a recipe it is best to buy unwaxed fruit. Alternatively, scrub the lemons with a brush, washing liquid and hot water, then rinse well.

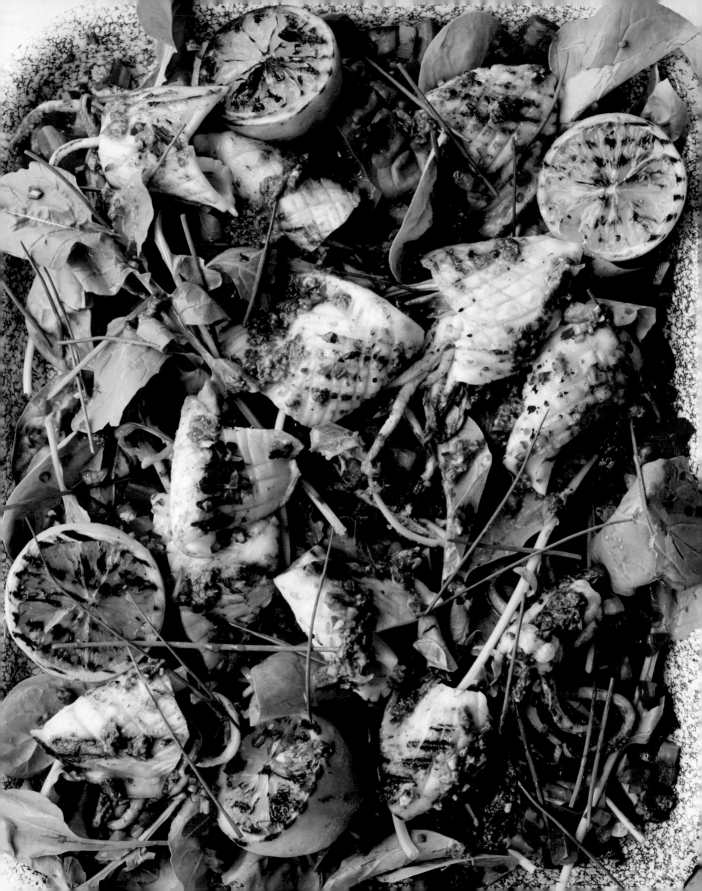

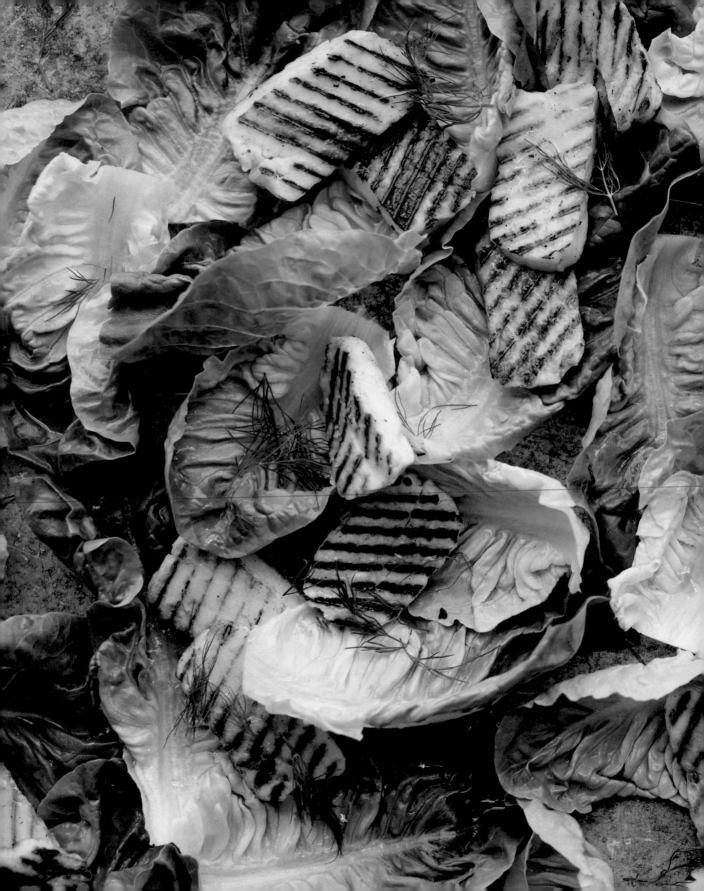

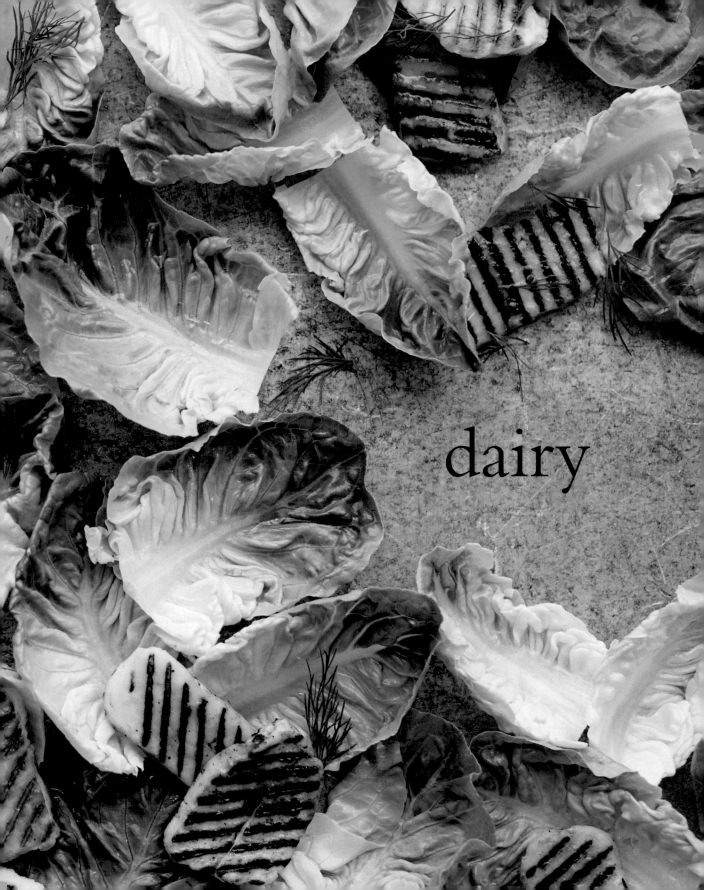

dairy

Ossau iraty is a French semi-hard sheep's cheese with a nutty taste and creamy texture that complements the earthy beetroot/beets. Use Parmesan, Gruyère or Emmental, if you prefer.

ossau iraty, asparagus & crouton salad

4 thick slices country-style bread, roughly torn into croutons
3 tablespoons olive oil
400 g/14 oz. asparagus spears, ends trimmed
150 g/5 oz. mixed baby salad leaves
4 raw chioggia beetroot/beets, cut into paper-thin round slices
100 g/3¾ oz. ossau iraty cheese, thinly sliced into shavings

DRESSING
6 tablespoons extra virgin olive oil
freshly squeezed juice of ½ small lemon
freshly squeezed juice of ½ small orange
1 teaspoon Dijon mustard
1 garlic clove, peeled and halved
salt and freshly ground black pepper

Serves 4

Preheat the oven to 200°C (400°F) Gas 6. While the oven is heating, put all the ingredients for the dressing in a small jar, season and shake until combined. Set aside.

Put the croutons in a small food bag and add 2 tablespoons of the oil. Shake the bag until the croutons are coated in the oil. Spread the croutons out evenly in a large roasting pan and toast in the preheated oven for 15 minutes, turning once, until golden and crisp.

Brush the remaining oil over the asparagus and season with salt and pepper. Arrange the asparagus in a separate roasting pan and roast, turning once, for 10 minutes until tender and just starting to colour.

Meanwhile, arrange the salad leaves on a large serving platter. Top with the beetroot/beets and asparagus, then spoon enough of the dressing over to coat and toss gently until combined. Sprinkle the ossau iraty and croutons over before serving.

Apple and cheese are natural partners. Here, the apples are pan-fried in a light honey-butter sauce until golden and glossy, while the piquant blue cheese balances out any sweetness.

Roquefort, pecan & apple salad

30 g/1 tablespoon butter
2 large, crisp eating apples, peeled, cored, and each apple cut into 10 wedges
1 tablespoon clear honey
100 g/3¾ oz. watercress, tough stalks removed
50 g/2 oz. baby spinach leaves, tough stalks discarded
175 g/6 oz. Roquefort or other blue cheese, crumbled into chunks

60 g/½ cup pecan halves, toasted

DRESSING
5 tablespoons extra virgin olive oil
2 tablespoons apple cider vinegar
1 teaspoon Dijon mustard
sea salt and freshly ground black pepper

Serves 4

Mix together all the ingredients for the dressing and season lightly with salt, bearing in mind that Roquefort cheese is quite salty, and more generously with pepper.

Melt the butter in a large, non-stick frying pan/skillet. Add the apple wedges and cook for 5 minutes, turning once. Stir in the honey, turn the apples to coat them in the honey-butter sauce and cook for 1 minute more, or until golden and glossy. Remove from the pan and set aside.

Spoon as much of the dressing over the watercress and spinach as needed to coat the leaves in a serving bowl. Toss until combined, then top with the apples, Roquefort cheese and pecans. Serve immediately.

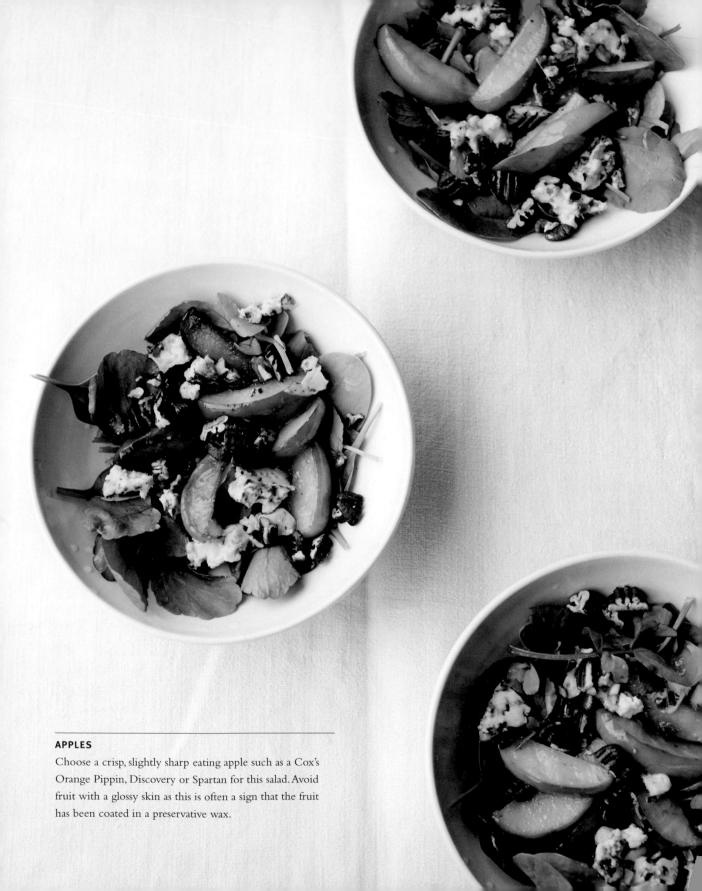

APPLES

Choose a crisp, slightly sharp eating apple such as a Cox's
Orange Pippin, Discovery or Spartan for this salad. Avoid
fruit with a glossy skin as this is often a sign that the fruit
has been coated in a preservative wax.

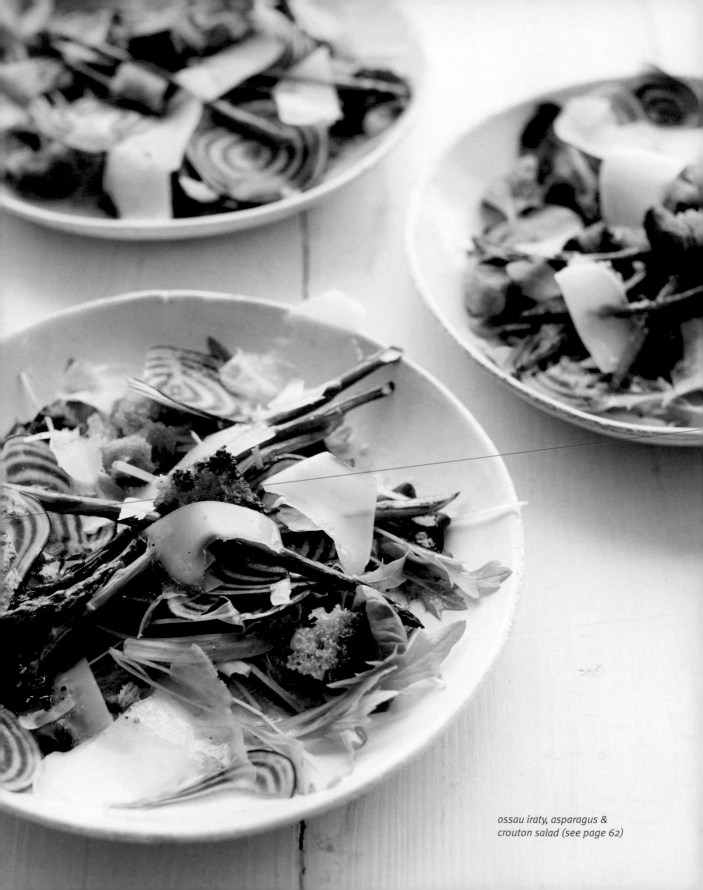

ossau iraty, asparagus & crouton salad (see page 62)

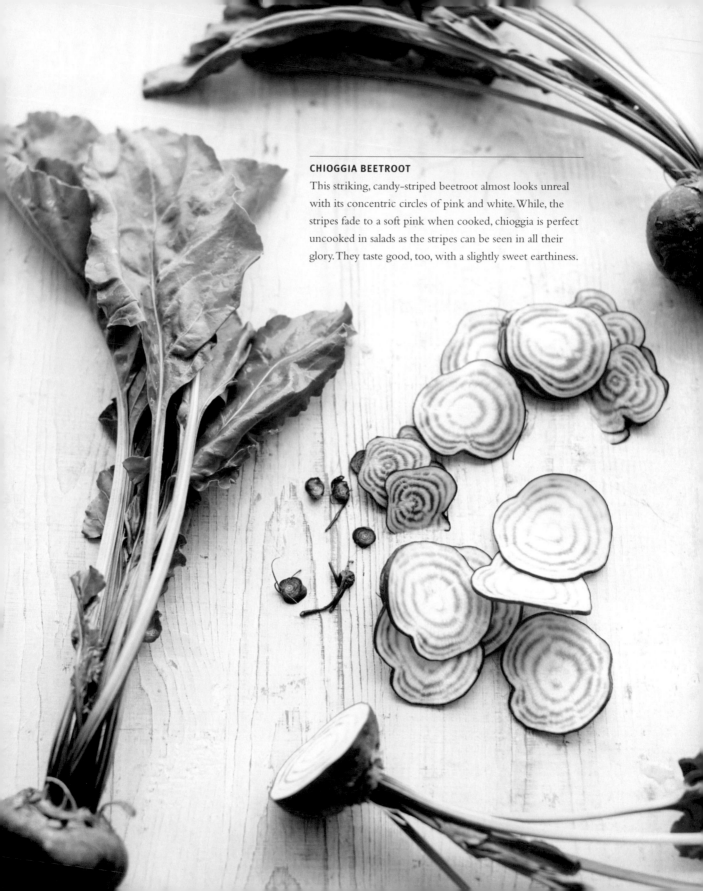

CHIOGGIA BEETROOT

This striking, candy-striped beetroot almost looks unreal with its concentric circles of pink and white. While, the stripes fade to a soft pink when cooked, chioggia is perfect uncooked in salads as the stripes can be seen in all their glory. They taste good, too, with a slightly sweet earthiness.

Full of the flavours of summer, this side dish would go well with poached salmon, roast chicken or griddled lamb steaks. If the chive stems are topped with their delicate purple flower heads, use them too, as they add both colour and flavour.

new potato, radish & chive salad with feta dressing

500 g/1 lb 2 oz. baby new potatoes, scrubbed and halved
100 g/3¾ oz. radishes, thinly sliced into rounds
½ cucumber, quartered, seeded and sliced
3 large handfuls of watercress, tough stems removed, torn into small sprigs
a handful of chives, including flowers if available

FETA DRESSING
150 g/5 oz. feta cheese, crumbled
125ml/½ cup natural/plain low-fat yogurt
freshly squeezed juice of 1 lemon
1 large garlic clove, crushed
2 large handfuls of mint leaves, finely chopped
sea salt and freshly ground black pepper

Serves 4

Cook the potatoes in plenty of boiling salted water for 12–15 minutes until tender, then drain and transfer to a large serving bowl.

Meanwhile, to make the dressing, blend the feta cheese, yogurt and lemon juice in a blender until smooth and creamy, then pour it into a bowl. Stir in the garlic and mint and season with pepper; you won't need any salt as the feta cheese is salty enough.

Add the radishes, cucumber and watercress to the bowl containing the potatoes. Snip half the chives over and add enough of the dressing to generously coat everything. Toss until thoroughly combined, and serve the salad with the remaining chives (and flowers, if any) arranged over the top.

YOGURT
Lower in fat and lighter than cream, yogurt adds a slightly tangy freshness to salad dressings. Look for a 'live' bio yogurt, which has had 'friendly bacteria' added to it.

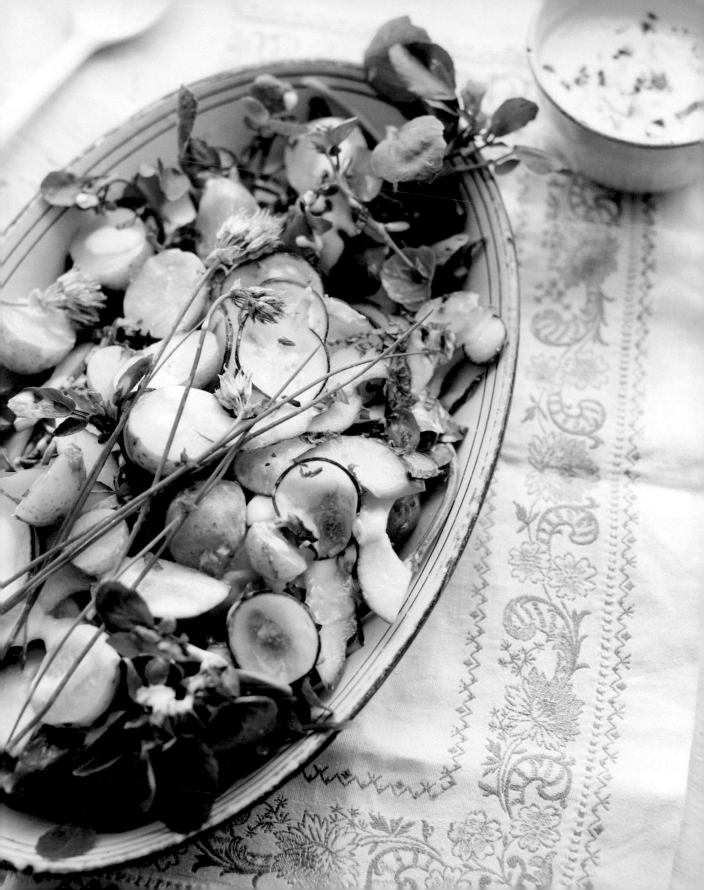

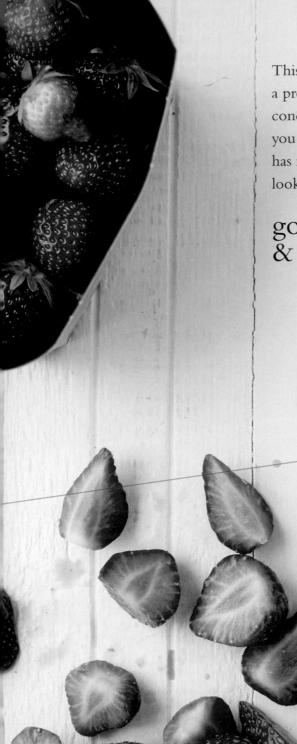

This sounds an unusual combination but it works… It is a pretty, fragrant and light salad, which makes the perfect conclusion to a meal on a hot summer's day, especially if you can't decide between dessert or cheese! Greek basil has much smaller leaves than regular and just suits the look of the dish, but you can use the latter if easier.

goat's cheese, strawberry & basil salad

350 g/12 oz. strawberries, hulled
150 g/5 oz. chevre blanc, crumbled
freshly squeezed juice of ½ lemon
1–2 tablespoons light olive oil

4 tablespoons Greek basil leaves
freshly ground black pepper

Serves 4

Halve or quarter the strawberries, if large, and arrange on a serving plate. Sprinkle the chevre blanc on top and squeeze the lemon juice over.

Drizzle with olive oil, sprinkle the basil leaves over and finish with a grinding of black pepper. Serve at room temperature.

STRAWBERRIES

Strawberries are available pretty much all year round nowadays, but nothing beats a strawberry bought in summer for its superior taste. For the best flavour, ensure the strawberry is at the peak of ripeness with no tough white or green parts.

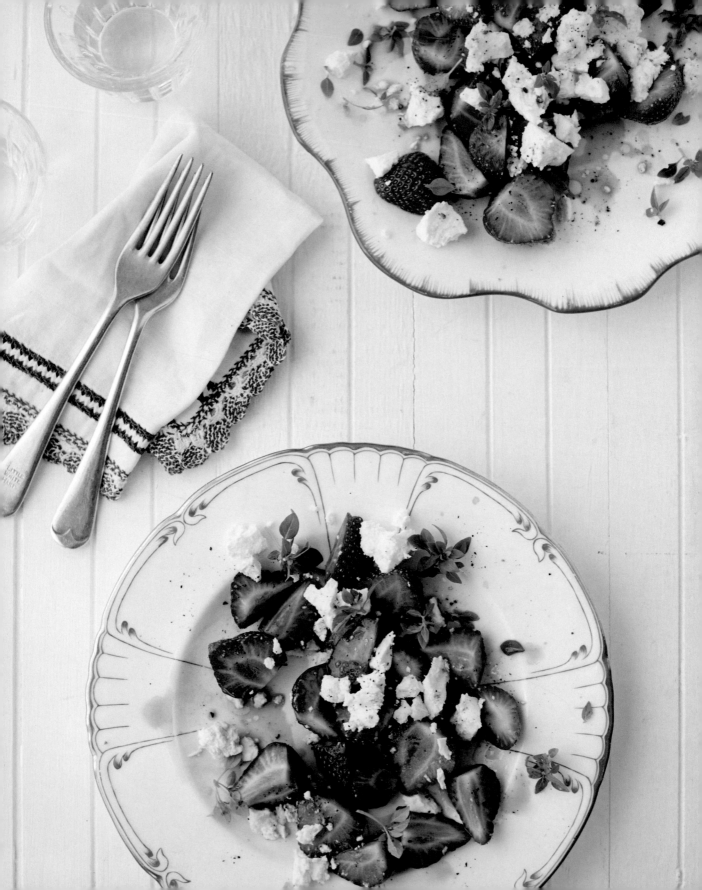

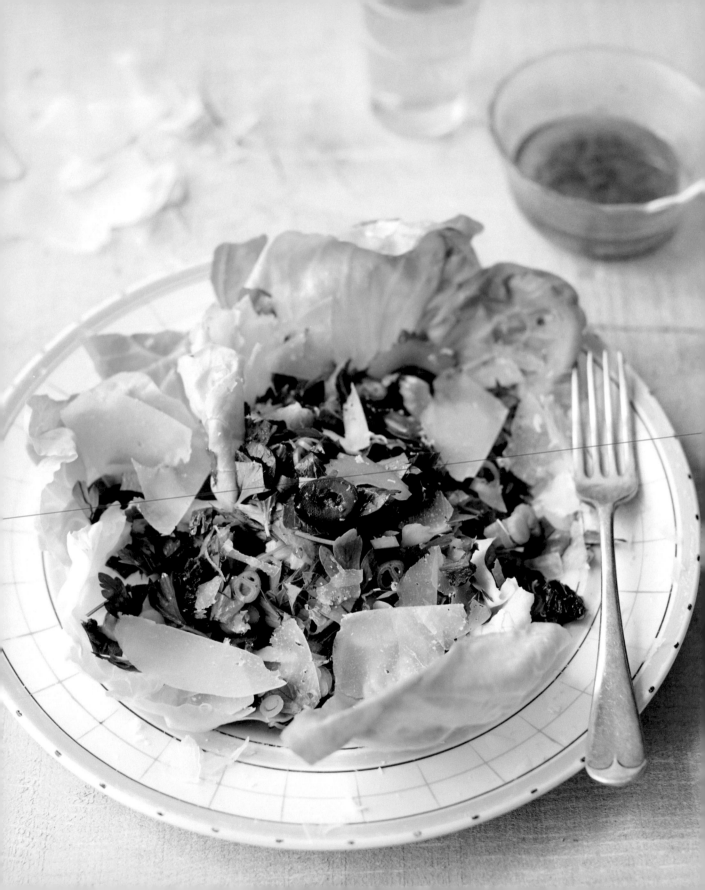

Fresh and vibrant, this robust salad makes an excellent accompaniment to fish, meat or egg dishes, and it's also good served on top of bruschetta or stirred into pasta, rice or beans. Pecorino works well, but so would a crumbly goat's cheese or a creamy burrata.

pecorino, olive & parsley salad

½ round/butterhead
    lettuce, leaves
    separated
6 large handfuls of
    freshly chopped flat
    leaf parsley
100 g/3¾ oz. pitted black
    olives, drained and
    thinly sliced into rounds
6 sun-dried tomatoes,
    finely chopped
3 celery sticks, finely
    chopped
3 spring onions/scallions,
    finely chopped
60 g/2¼ oz. Pecorino
    cheese, sliced into thin
    shavings

DRESSING
4 tablespoons extra
    virgin olive oil
finely grated zest and
    freshly squeezed juice
    of 1 lemon
2 teaspoons red wine
    vinegar
1 small garlic clove,
    crushed
sea salt and freshly
    ground black pepper

Serves 4

Arrange the lettuce leaves in a salad bowl. Combine the parsley, olives, sun-dried tomatoes, celery and spring onions/scallions in a separate bowl.

Mix together all the ingredients for the dressing and season. Pour enough of the dressing over the parsley mixture to coat, and toss until combined. Spoon the mixture on top of the lettuce leaves, then sprinkle the Pecorino cheese over before serving.

The goat's cheese is baked until soft and unctuous, and when served on top of the beetroot/beets salad it makes a perfect light meal or appetizer with slices of country-style bread.

baked goat's cheese with honey-spiced beetroot

8 baby uncooked
    beetroot/beets,
    washed and trimmed
1 tablespoon clear honey
1 teaspoon harissa
    spice mix
100 g/3¾ oz. rocket/
    arugula leaves
60 g/⅓ cup pea shoots
2 red chicory/Belgian
    endive heads, sliced
4 tablespoons freshly
    snipped chives

4 x 100 g/3¾ oz. English
    goat's cheeses, halved
    horizontally

DRESSING
5 tablespoons extra
    virgin olive oil
1 tablespoon balsamic
    vinegar
sea salt and freshly
    ground black pepper

Serves 4

Preheat the oven to 200°C (400°F) Gas 6. Brush the beetroot/beets with 1 tablespoon of the oil and roast for 30 minutes until almost tender. Mix together the honey and harissa with another tablespoon of the oil in a bowl, then season. Transfer the beetroot/beets to the bowl and turn until coated in the honey spice mix. Return the beetroot/beets to the roasting pan and roast for another 10 minutes or until tender.

Meanwhile, mix together all the ingredients for the dressing and season. Arrange the rocket/arugula, pea shoots, chicory/Belgian endive and chives on 4 plates.

Just before the beetroot/beets are ready, place the goat's cheese halves in a second roasting pan, skin-side down. Bake for 5 minutes until soft and starting to run.

Slice the beetroot/beets into quarters and arrange on top of the salad portions, drizzle the dressing over and top each portion with 2 halves of goat's cheese.

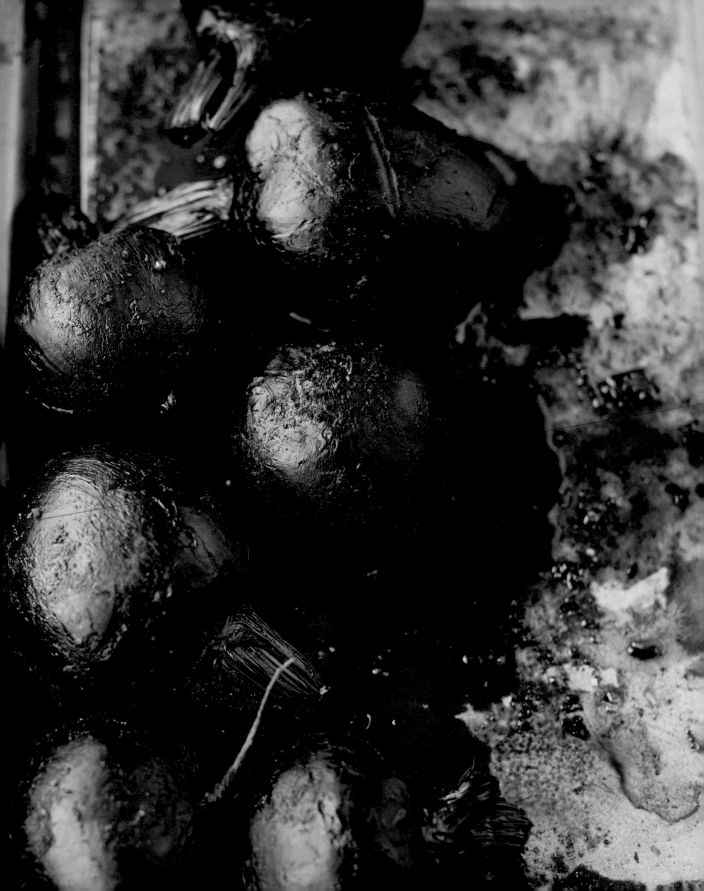

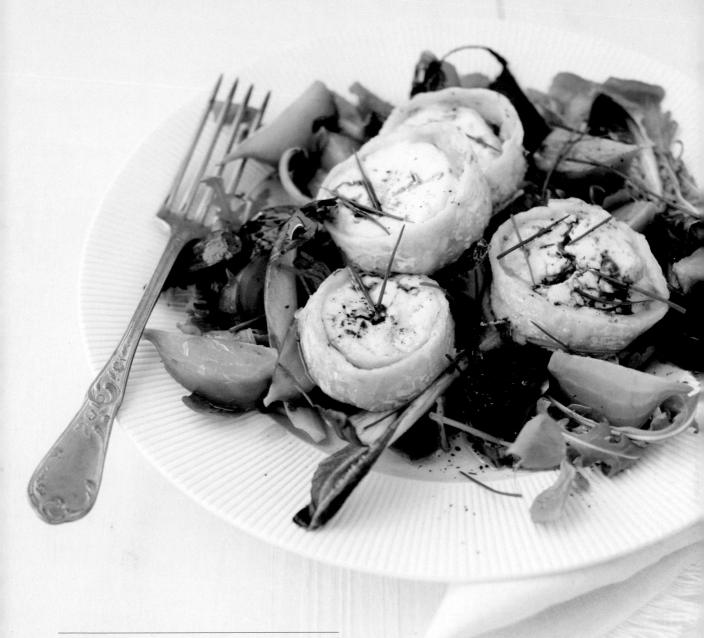

BEETROOT

Beetroot/beets become sweet and almost caramelized when roasted, and its natural earthiness is lifted by the honey and harissa spices in this recipe. Experiment with different varieties, such as golden beetroot/beets.

baked goat's cheese with honey-
spiced beetroot (see page 71)

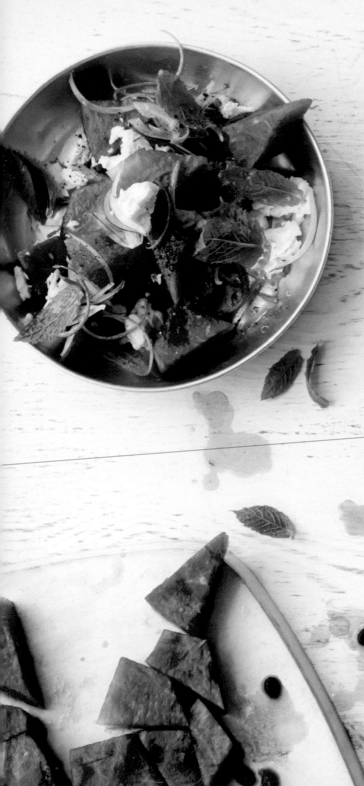

A firm favourite – you can't beat the combination of salty, crumbly feta cheese with sweet, juicy watermelon and the zing of fresh lime.

feta, watermelon & lime salad

½ small watermelon
250 g/9 oz. feta cheese, cut into bite-sized cubes
½ small red onion, thinly sliced
freshly squeezed juice of 1 lime
extra virgin olive oil, for drizzling

pared zest of ¼ lime, cut into fine strips
a generous handful of mint leaves
freshly ground black pepper

Serves 4

Slice the watermelon away from the skin, remove any seeds and cut into bite-sized cubes; you should have about 500 g/1 lb 2 oz. of fruit.

Divide the watermelon between 4 serving plates and top with the feta cheese and red onion. Squeeze the lime juice over and drizzle with a little olive oil. Garnish with the lime zest and mint leaves, and season with black pepper.

WATERMELON

Despite watermelon's high water content, it is particularly rich in vitamins A and C. Nutritional benefits aside, you really can't beat its incredible colour and sweet juiciness.

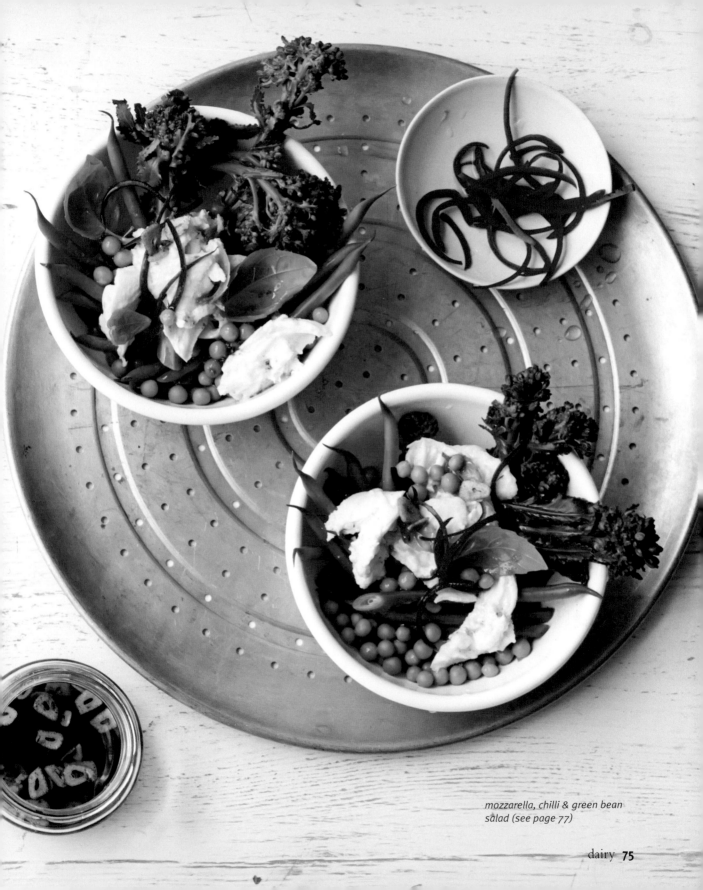

mozzarella, chilli & green bean
salad (see page 77)

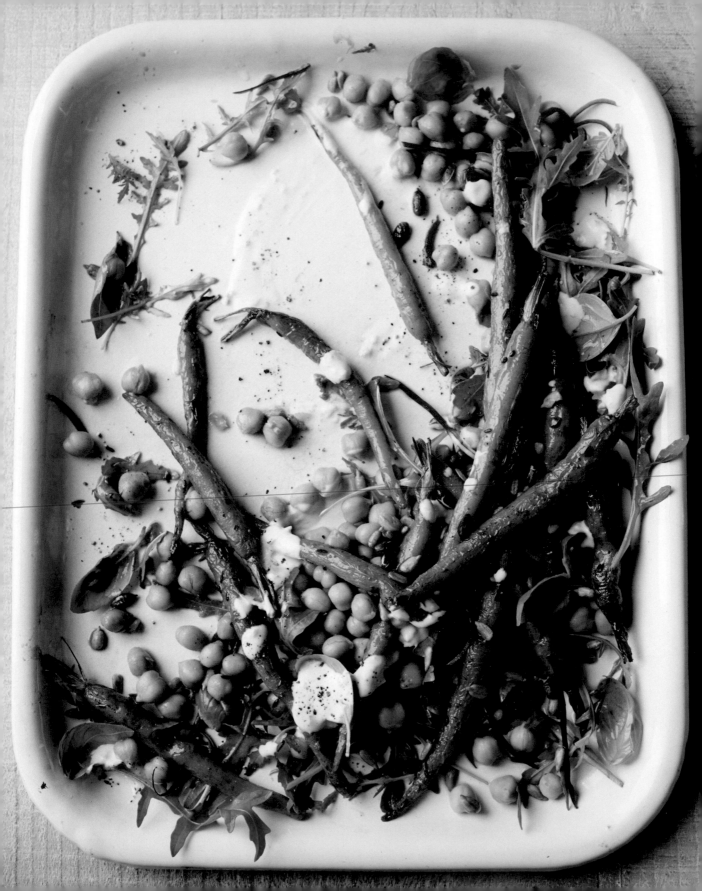

Sweet, sticky and spicy, here carrots are combined with chickpeas and toasted seeds, and served with a fragrant cream made with fresh orange zest and juice mixed with crème fraîche.

honey-roasted carrots & seeds with citrus cream

600 g/1lb. 5oz. baby
   carrots, scrubbed
   and trimmed
3 tablespoons extra
   virgin olive oil, plus
   extra for drizzling
2 tablespoons balsamic
   vinegar
1 teaspoon cumin seeds
2 teaspoons clear honey
400 g/14 oz. canned
   chickpeas, drained
   and rinsed
2 large handfuls of
   rocket/arugula leaves
1 red chilli/chile, seeded
   and thinly sliced

2 handfuls of basil leaves
4 tablespoons mixed
   sunflower and pumpkin
   seeds, toasted
sea salt and freshly
   ground black pepper

CITRUS CREAM
100 ml/⅓ cup crème
   fraîche
finely grated zest
   of ½ orange
3 tablespoons freshly
   squeezed orange juice

Serves 4

Preheat the oven to 200°C (400°F) Gas 6. Put the carrots in a large roasting pan and drizzle over enough oil to coat, season, then toss them with your hands. Roast the carrots for 15 minutes, then stir in the balsamic vinegar and sprinkle the cumin seeds over. Return the carrots to the oven for another 15 minutes or until tender and starting to turn golden.

   Meanwhile, for the citrus cream mix together the crème fraîche, the orange zest and half the juice in a bowl.

   Transfer the carrots to a bowl. Stir the honey and remaining orange juice into the juices in the roasting pan until combined and then pour over the carrots. Add the chickpeas, rocket/arugula and chilli/chile and toss until mixed together. Divide between 4 serving plates and arrange the basil leaves and toasted seeds over. Top each serving with a spoonful of the citrus cream.

The heat of the chilli/chile as well as the garlicky anchovy dressing are tempered by the mild creaminess of the mozzarella and slight sweetness of the green vegetables in this simple summery salad.

mozzarella, chilli & green bean salad

200 g/7 oz. green beans,
   trimmed
200 g/7 oz. long-stem
   broccoli, trimmed
100 g/1 cup shelled peas,
   or frozen garden peas,
   defrosted
2 x 125-g/4¼-oz. balls
   mozzarella, drained,
   patted dry and torn
   into pieces
1 red chilli/chile, seeded
   and thinly sliced
a generous handful of
   basil leaves, torn
sea salt and freshly
   ground black pepper

DRESSING
5 tablespoons extra
   virgin olive oil
2 large garlic cloves,
   sliced
2 anchovy fillets in oil,
   drained and chopped
freshly squeezed juice
   of ½ lemon

Serves 4

Steam the green beans, broccoli and peas until just tender, then refresh briefly under cold running water so the vegetables remain warm.

   Meanwhile, for the dressing heat the olive oil, garlic and anchovies gently in a small pan, stirring and mashing the anchovies against the side of the pan to encourage them to melt into the oil. Heat for 4 minutes until the garlic starts to colour. Stir in the lemon juice.

   Arrange the vegetables on a large serving plate and top with the mozzarella and chilli/chile. Spoon enough of the dressing over to coat and toss gently. Sprinkle with basil leaves and check the seasoning, adding salt and pepper if needed.

Pomegranate molasses, a popular ingredient in Middle Eastern cooking, lends a tangy, sweet-sour flavour to the dressing for this main meal salad. It also makes a useful base for a marinade and goes particularly well with bean, poultry, meat and vegetable dishes.

char-grilled halloumi, courgette & mint salad

125 g/4 oz. rocket/
    arugula leaves
600 g/1lb. 5oz. canned
    chickpeas, drained
    and rinsed
1 small red onion, sliced
1 courgette/zucchini,
    coarsely grated
400 g/14 oz. halloumi,
    patted dry and sliced
seeds from ½
    pomegranate
4 tablespoons freshly
    chopped mint leaves

**POMEGRANATE
MOLASSES DRESSING**
4 tablespoons extra
    virgin olive oil, plus
    extra for brushing
2 tablespoons
    pomegranate molasses
1 teaspoon freshly
    squeezed lemon juice
½ teaspoon caster/
    superfine sugar
sea salt and freshly
    ground black pepper

Serves 4

Mix together all the ingredients for the dressing and season with salt and pepper.

Divide the rocket/arugula, chickpeas, red onion and courgette/zucchini between 4 serving plates. Spoon enough of the dressing over the salad to lightly coat it and toss gently until everything is combined.

Heat a large, ridged griddle pan over a high heat. Brush the halloumi slices with a little extra olive oil. Reduce the heat a little and griddle the halloumi for 2 minutes on each side or until slightly blackened in places and softened. Serve the halloumi on top of the salad, garnished with the pomegranate seeds and mint.

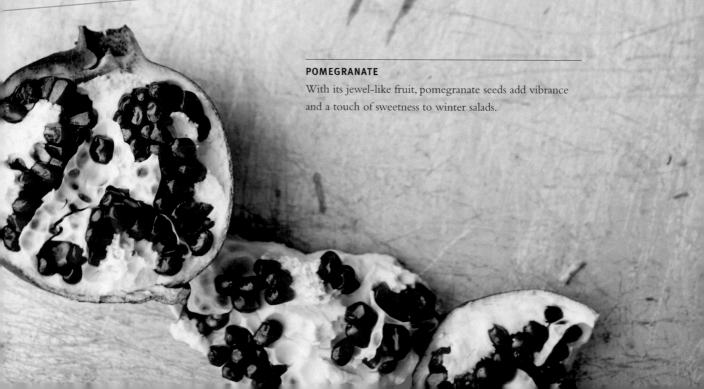

POMEGRANATE
With its jewel-like fruit, pomegranate seeds add vibrance and a touch of sweetness to winter salads.

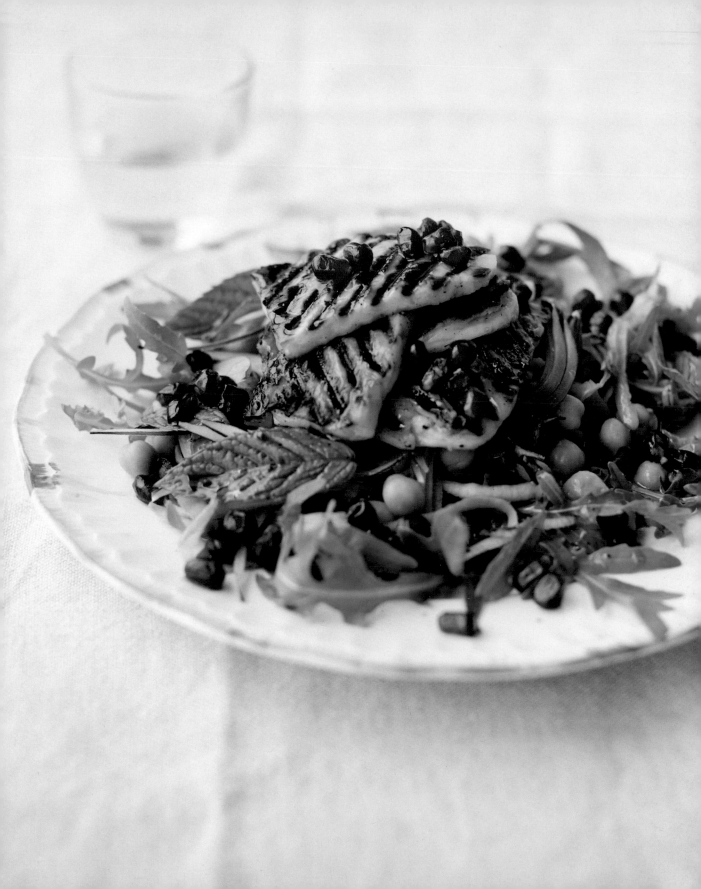

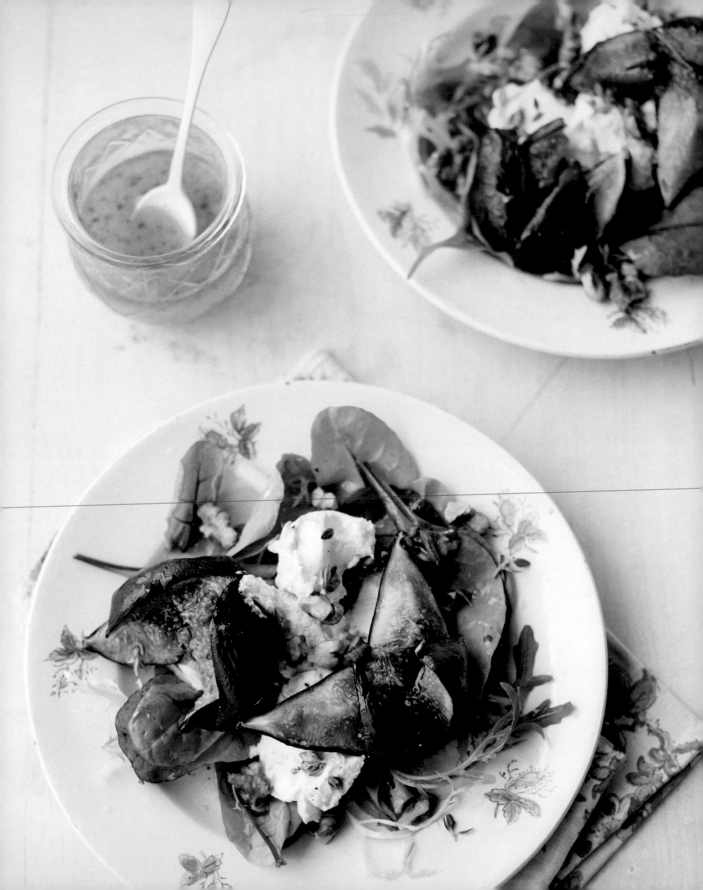

Try your hand at cheesemaking with this main-meal salad. Labneh is an easy-to-make Middle Eastern drained yogurt cheese, and is similar in consistency to a thick cream cheese or curd/farmer's cheese. Its mild fresh flavour combines beautifully with the sticky honey-coated figs and toasted walnuts.

labneh with honey-roasted figs & walnuts

8 large ripe figs
2 tablespoons clear
  honey
125 g/4¼ oz. mixed soft,
  baby salad leaves
50 g/2 oz. walnut pieces,
  toasted
2 tablespoons lemon
  thyme leaves, oregano
  or basil

LABNEH
350 g/12 oz. good-quality
  Greek/US strained
  plain yogurt or thick
  natural/plain yogurt
1 teaspoon sea salt

DRESSING
2 tablespoons freshly
  squeezed lemon juice
1 tablespoon freshly
  squeezed orange juice
5 tablespoons extra
  virgin olive oil
freshly ground black
  pepper

Serves 4

First, to make the labneh, rest a sieve/strainer over a medium mixing bowl and line it with a double layer of cheesecloth, muslin or a kitchen cloth that is large enough to overhang the sides.

Mix the yogurt with the salt and pour it into the cloth-lined sieve/strainer. Pull the cloth up around the yogurt and twist the top to make a bundle. Leave the yogurt to drain in the fridge for at least 12 hours or up to 24 hours; the longer you leave it, the firmer the labneh will be.

Thirty minutes before you want to serve the salad, preheat the oven to 190°C (375°F) Gas 5.

Cut a deep cross down into the pointed top of each fig, nearly to the bottom, then squeeze the sides slightly to open it out. Place the figs in a roasting dish and drizzle over three-quarters of the honey. Roast for 15 minutes or until glossy and tender, spooning over any honey in the bottom of the dish halfway through.

Remove the cheesecloth bundle from the sieve/strainer and open it to reveal a smooth, thick round of soft cheese. Crumble two-thirds of it into large bite-sized pieces (the remaining labneh will keep in the refrigerator in an airtight container for up to 3 days).

Arrange the salad leaves on a serving plate. For the dressing, mix together the citrus juices, olive oil and the remaining honey. Season, and drizzle half of the dressing over the leaves, then gently toss until combined. Top with the figs, labneh and toasted walnuts, drizzle with the remaining dressing and sprinkle with the lemon thyme before serving.

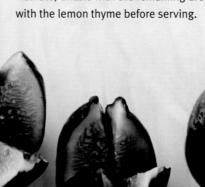

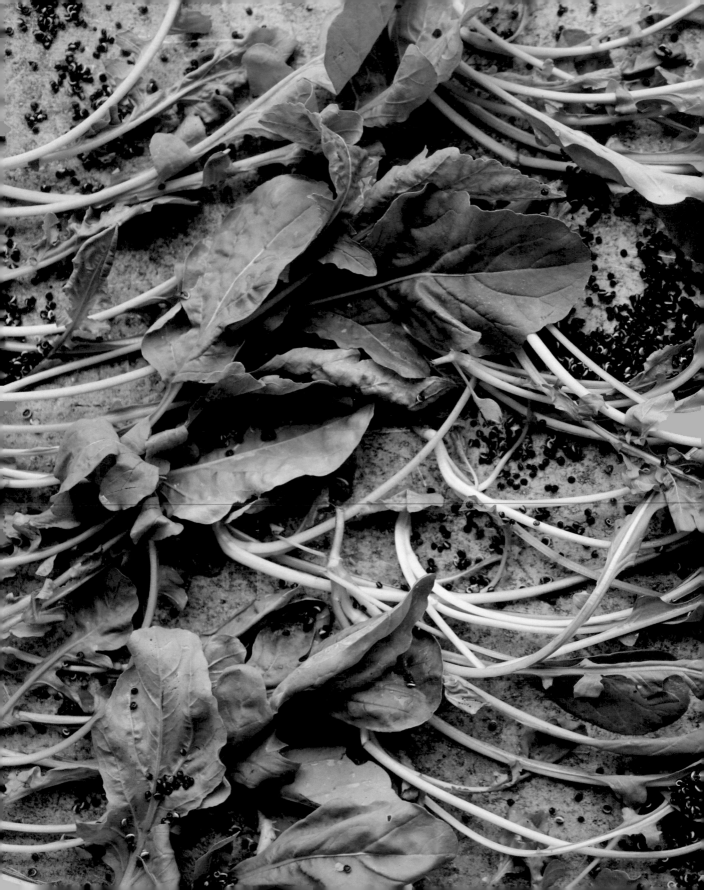

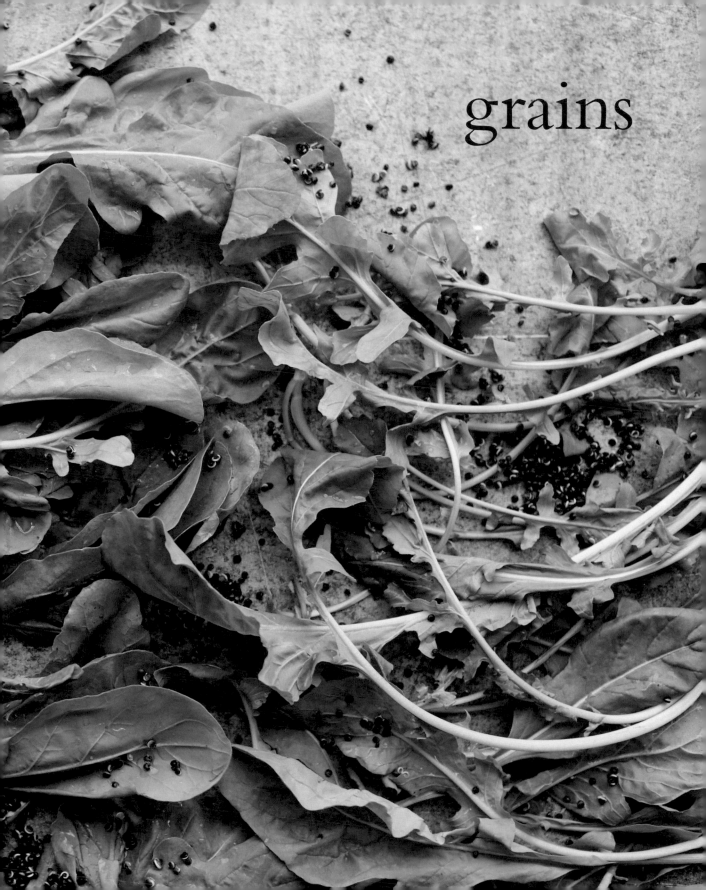

grains

A rustic, warming, wintry dish, this salad is both hearty and sustaining. Pearl barley has a slightly chewy texture when cooked and goes well with strong flavours, such as rosemary, garlic and smoked Cheddar cheese as in this recipe. The salad is also good topped with shards of crispy bacon.

warm pearl barley, smoked Cheddar & walnut salad

200 g/7 oz. pearl barley, rinsed
60 g/½ cup walnut pieces
1 large onion, chopped
3 cloves garlic, finely chopped
1 tablespoon freshly chopped rosemary
400 g/14 oz. baby spinach leaves, sliced
2 handfuls of freshly chopped flat leaf parsley
100 g/3¾ oz. smoked Cheddar cheese, cut into small cubes

DRESSING
4 tablespoons extra virgin olive oil
1 heaped teaspoon wholegrain mustard
1 heaped teaspoon clear honey
freshly squeezed juice of 1 lemon
sea salt and freshly ground black pepper

Serves 4

Put the barley in a medium-sized pan and cover generously with water. Bring to the boil, then turn the heat down and simmer, part-covered, for 30 minutes or until tender. Drain and set aside.

Meanwhile, toast the walnuts in a large, dry sauté pan for 4 minutes, turning occasionally, until they smell toasted and start to colour. Transfer to a bowl and leave to cool.

Add 2 tablespoons of the olive oil to the sauté pan and fry the onion for 6 minutes, stirring regularly, until softened. Add the garlic, rosemary and spinach, and cook for another 3 minutes, turning the leaves with tongs, until the spinach has wilted.

Meanwhile, mix all the ingredients for the dressing together until combined, and season with salt and pepper.

Transfer the barley to a serving bowl with the spinach mixture and parsley. Pour the dressing over and toss until combined. Add the Cheddar cheese cubes and toss again, then serve, sprinkled with the walnuts.

PEARL BARLEY
An underrated and economical alternative to rice, pearl barley is the perfect comfort food with its soft, slightly nutty grain. Pearl barley cooks more quickly than pot barley as it has had its outer bran and husk removed, but they are interchangeable in this recipe.

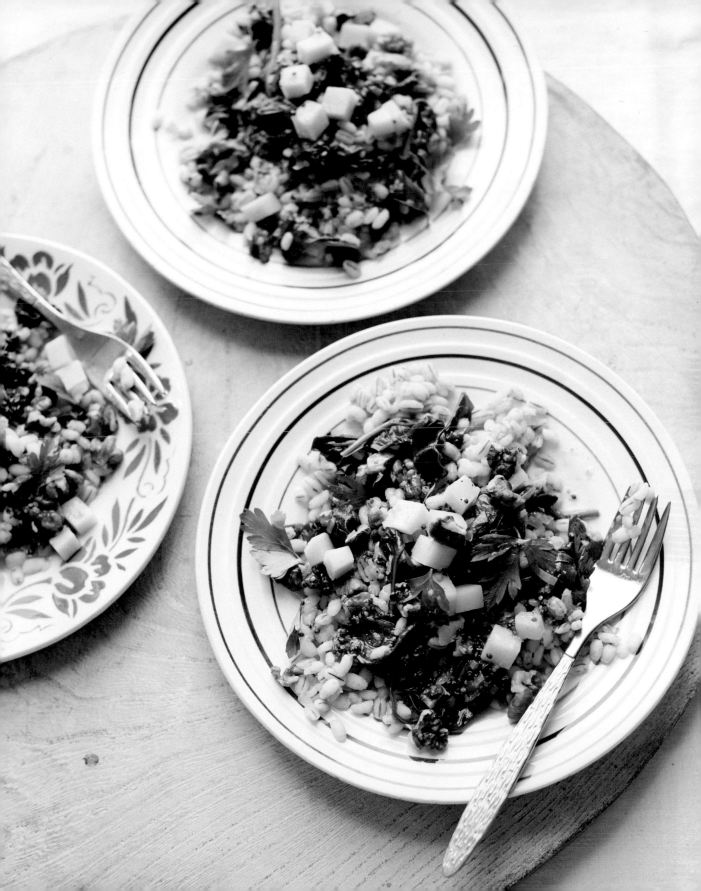

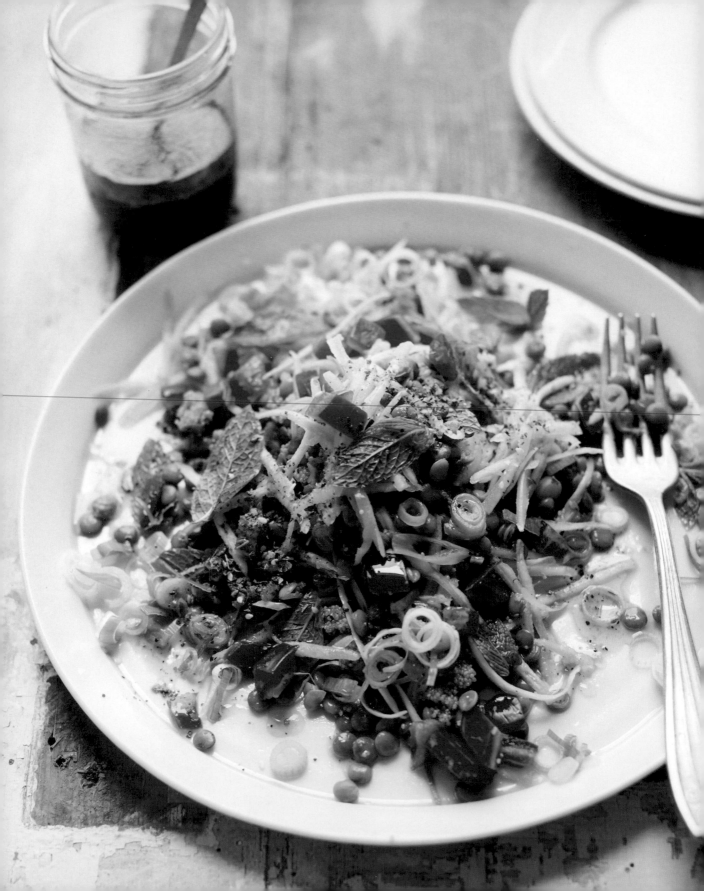

This tiny grain (or, more accurately, seed) packs a powerful nutritional punch for its diminutive size. Popular in South America, amaranth is gluten-free as well as being a good source of digestible protein and valuable minerals. I find it is best mixed with other grains or pulses to give it a bit more substance.

amaranth & green lentil salad with za'atar

165 g/5½ oz. green
    lentils, rinsed
4 tablespoons amaranth
6 spring onions/
    scallions, thinly sliced
6 vine-ripened tomatoes,
    roughly chopped
1 yellow courgette/
    zucchini, coarsely
    grated
2 handfuls of freshly
    chopped mint leaves,
    plus a few whole
    leaves to decorate
1 tablespoon za'atar
    (see page 11)

DRESSING
2 tablespoons
    pomegranate molasses
3 tablespoons extra
    virgin olive oil
finely grated zest and
    freshly squeezed juice
    of 1 lemon
sea salt and freshly
    ground black pepper

Serves 4

Put the lentils in a large pan and cover with plenty of cold water. Bring to the boil, then turn the heat down and simmer, part-covered, for 20 minutes or until tender. Drain and transfer the lentils to a serving bowl.

Meanwhile, toast the amaranth in a dry pan for 2 minutes, shaking the pan regularly, until the grains start to pop and turn golden. Pour enough water over to cover and bring to the boil, then turn the heat down and simmer for 6 minutes or until tender. Drain and add to the bowl with the lentils.

Mix together all the dressing ingredients and season.

Add the spring onions/scallions, tomatoes, courgette/zucchini and mint to the serving bowl, and pour enough of the dressing over to coat. Toss until combined and serve, sprinkled with the za'atar and a few whole mint leaves.

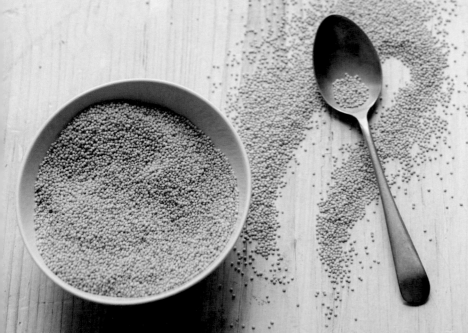

freekeh, pumpkin & crispy ginger salad

Like quinoa, freekeh is rich in protein and has a slightly nutty, earthy flavour, but you can use quinoa instead, or even bulghur wheat. Middle Eastern in origin, freekeh is a green wheat that is picked unripe and then roasted to give it a slight smokiness.

500 g/1 lb 2 oz. pumpkin
  or butternut squash,
  skin removed, seeded
  and cut into pieces
3 tablespoons olive oil
125 g/1 cup freekeh
3-cm/1¼-in. piece fresh
  root ginger, peeled and
  cut into thin strips
1 large onion, chopped
2 large garlic cloves,
  chopped
3 handfuls of sultanas/
  golden raisins

finely grated zest and
  freshly squeezed juice
  of 1 orange
1 teaspoon ground allspice
1 teaspoon ground ginger
squeeze of lemon juice
2 handfuls of freshly
  chopped coriander/
  cilantro leaves, plus
  a few whole leaves
  to decorate
sea salt and freshly
  ground black pepper

Serves 4

Preheat the oven to 200°C (400°F) Gas 6. Toss the pumpkin in 1 tablespoon of the oil and season, then spread out evenly in a large roasting pan. Roast for 30–35 minutes, turning once, until tender and starting to turn golden in places.

Meanwhile, put the freekeh in a pan and cover with water. Bring to the boil, then turn the heat down, cover and simmer for 15 minutes or until tender. Drain and transfer to a serving bowl.

Heat the remaining oil in a frying pan/skillet over a medium heat and fry the ginger for 3 minutes, until crisp and golden. Remove from the pan with a slotted spoon, drain on paper towels and set aside. Add the onion to the pan and fry for 8 minutes, stirring regularly, until softened. Add the garlic and cook for a further minute.

Stir the onion and garlic into the freekeh with the sultanas/golden raisins, orange zest and juice, allspice and ginger. Add a squeeze of lemon juice and the coriander/cilantro, season well, and stir until combined. Serve, sprinkled with the crispy ginger.

Quinoa makes a nutritious alternative to the more usual bulghur wheat in a tabbouleh. The secret to a successful tabbouleh is to get the right balance of grain to fresh produce; too much of the former makes for a slightly dull salad so be generous with the herbs and vegetables.

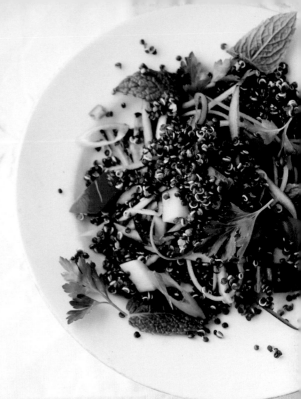

red quinoa tabbouleh

125 g/4¼ oz. red quinoa
6 vine-ripened tomatoes, quartered, seeded and chopped
2 small Lebanese cucumbers, quartered lengthways and diced
4 spring onions/scallions, finely chopped
1 courgette/zucchini, coarsely grated
6 tablespoons freshly chopped mint
6 tablespoons freshly chopped flat leaf parsley

DRESSING
3 tablespoons extra virgin olive oil
4 tablespoons freshly squeezed lemon juice
a pinch of cumin seeds
sea salt and freshly ground black pepper

Serves 4

Put the quinoa in a pan and cover with water. Bring to the boil, then turn the heat down and simmer, covered, for 10–15 minutes until tender. Drain, transfer the quinoa to a serving bowl and leave to cool slightly.

Meanwhile, mix together all the ingredients for the dressing and season to taste.

Add the tomatoes, cucumbers, spring onions/scallions, courgette/zucchini and herbs to the quinoa. Pour the dressing over and toss to combine everything. Check the seasoning and serve at room temperature.

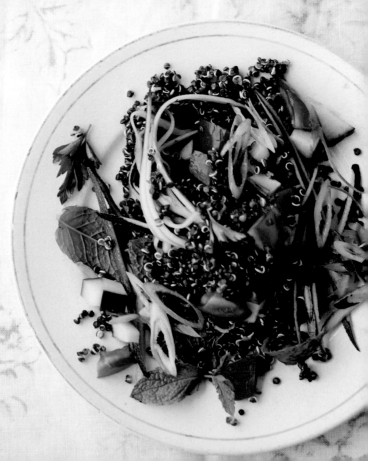

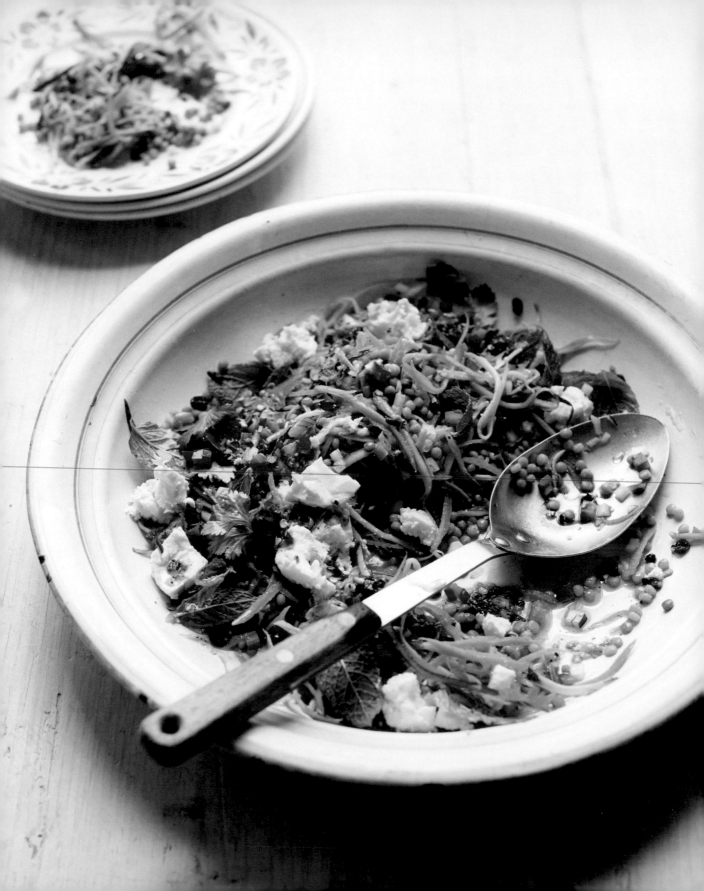

In keeping with the North African feel, the giant couscous is flavoured with berberries, small, slightly sweet-sour red berries, which can be swapped with dried sour cherries, cranberries or raisins, if you like.

golden spiced giant couscous

125 g/4¼ oz. giant
    wholemeal couscous
    or mograbiah
1 teaspoon ground
    turmeric
2 carrots, coarsely grated
1 courgette/zucchini,
    coarsely grated
1 red onion, finely
    chopped
1 large red (bell) pepper
    pepper, seeded
    and diced
2 handfuls of berberries,
    dried sour cherries,
    cranberries or raisins
2 large handfuls of freshly
    chopped mint leaves
2 large handfuls of freshly
    chopped coriander/
    cilantro leaves
100 g/3¾ oz. feta
    cheese, crumbled

DRESSING
4 tablespoons extra
    virgin olive oil
finely grated zest and
    freshly squeezed juice
    of 2 lemons
½ teaspoon dried chilli
    flakes/hot pepper
    flakes
1 teaspoon coriander
    seeds, toasted and
    ground
sea salt and freshly
    ground black pepper

Serves 4

Put the giant couscous in a pan and cover with water, stir in the turmeric and some salt, and bring to the boil. Reduce the heat and simmer, covered, for 6–8 minutes or until tender. Drain and transfer to a serving bowl.

Meanwhile, mix together all the ingredients for the dressing and season.

Add the carrots, courgette/zucchini, onion, red pepper/bell pepper, berberries and herbs to the giant couscous and pour the dressing over. Toss until combined and serve topped with crumbled feta cheese.

GIANT COUSCOUS

The intriguingly named 'giant couscous' also goes by the name 'mograbieh'. The rolled balls of semolina are simply couscous but in a larger form, so they lend a little more substance to a dish, but still have a soft, yielding texture when cooked.

Orzo, the small, rice-shaped pasta also known as risoni, is perfect for salads as it holds its shape when cooked and combines beautifully with other ingredients. Serve this orzo salad on its own or as an accompaniment to grilled meat, fish or vegetables.

Kamut, or khorasan wheat, is an ancient type of Middle Eastern wheat, which is experiencing a resurgence in popularity. This high-protein grain has a nutty flavour and keeps its texture after cooking, but you can use barley or rice instead, if you cannot get hold of it.

orzo & roasted tomatoes with pesto dressing

400 g/14 oz. vine-ripened cherry tomatoes
250 g/9 oz. dried orzo
100 g/3¾ oz. rocket/arugula leaves
2 handfuls of basil leaves
6 tablespoons pine nuts, toasted
50 g/2 oz. Parmesan cheese shavings

PESTO DRESSING
6 heaped tablespoons basil pesto
2 tablespoons extra virgin olive oil, plus extra for drizzling
sea salt and freshly ground black pepper

Serves 4

Preheat the oven to 220°C (425°F) Gas 7. Put the tomatoes in a roasting pan and drizzle over a little olive oil, turn to coat them in the oil, season and roast in the preheated oven for 20 minutes until softened and starting to colour.

Meanwhile, cook the orzo in a large pan of boiling salted water following the pack instructions, then drain, reserving 2 tablespoons of the cooking water. Put the orzo into a serving bowl.

Mix together all the ingredients for the pesto dressing, stir in the reserved cooking water and season. Spoon the dressing over the orzo and stir until combined. Add the roasted tomatoes and rocket/arugula and toss again gently. Garnish with the basil, pine nuts and Parmesan cheese before serving.

kamut with chermoula dressing

400 g/14 oz. vine-ripened cherry tomatoes
1 tablespoon extra virgin olive oil
150 g/5 oz. kamut
200 g/7 oz. spring greens/collards or kale, tough outer leaves and stems discarded, leaves finely shredded
2 large handfuls of coriander/cilantro leaves, chopped

CHERMOULA DRESSING
1 small preserved lemon and 2 tablespoons juice from the jar
4 tablespoons extra virgin olive oil
2 garlic cloves, crushed
1 teaspoon each ground cumin, ground ginger and ground coriander
½ teaspoon dried chilli flakes/hot pepper flakes
sea salt and freshly ground black pepper

Serves 4

Preheat the oven to 200°C (400°F) Gas 6. Toss the tomatoes in the oil and spread out in a large roasting pan. Roast for 15–20 minutes, until starting to collapse.

Meanwhile, put the kamut in a pan and cover with plenty of water. Bring to the boil, then turn the heat down, part-cover and simmer for 10–12 minutes, until tender. Drain and transfer to a serving bowl with the spring greens/collards and coriander/cilantro.

For the dressing, scoop out and discard the flesh from the preserved lemon. Finely chop the skin and combine it with the rest of the ingredients in a bowl. Season. Spoon half of the dressing over the salad and toss to combine. Pile the tomatoes on top, then spoon over the rest of the dressing and serve.

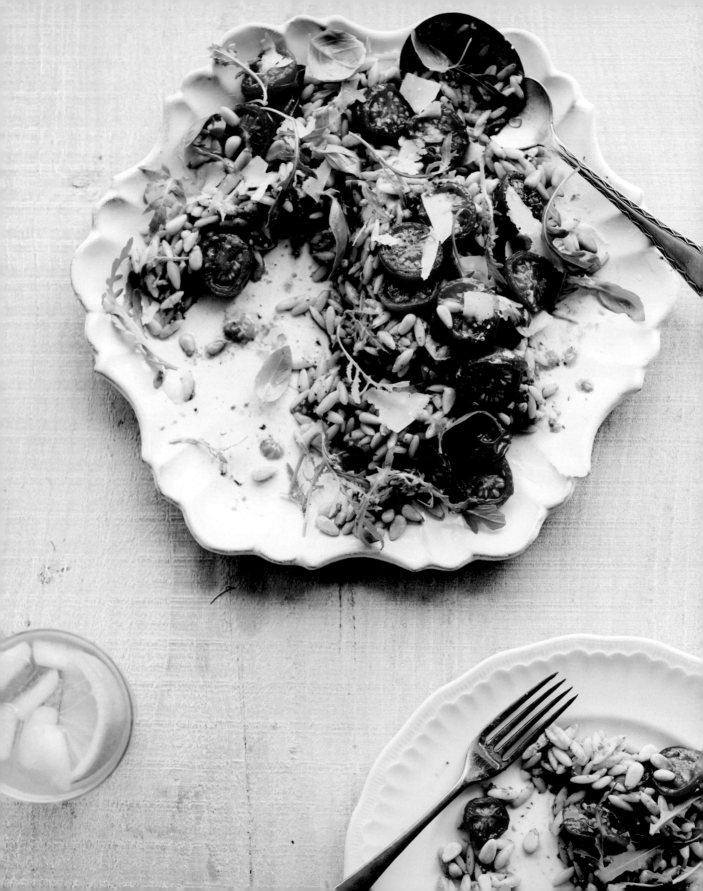

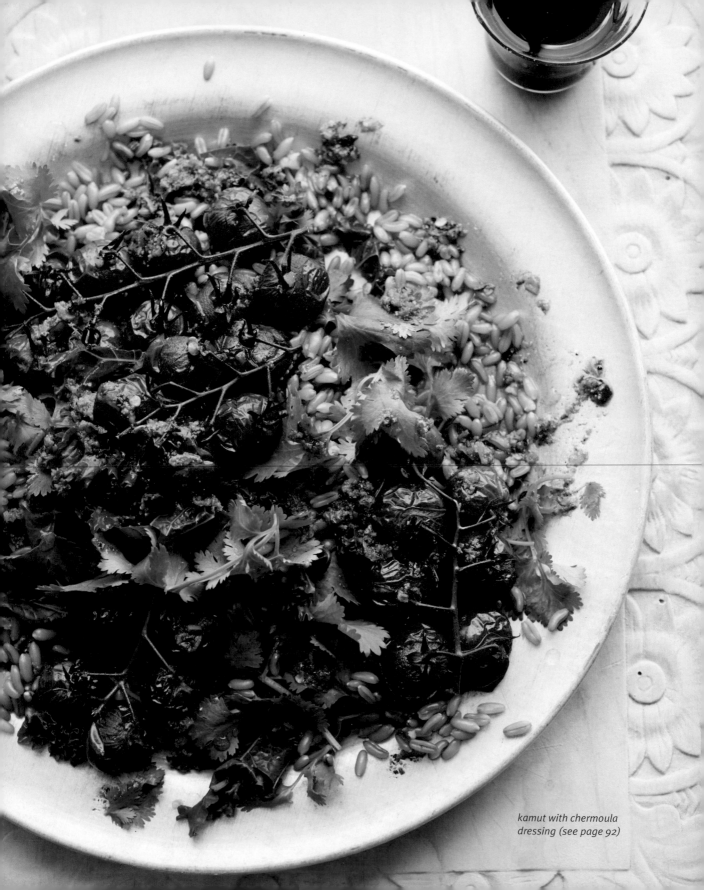

kamut with chermoula dressing (see page 92)

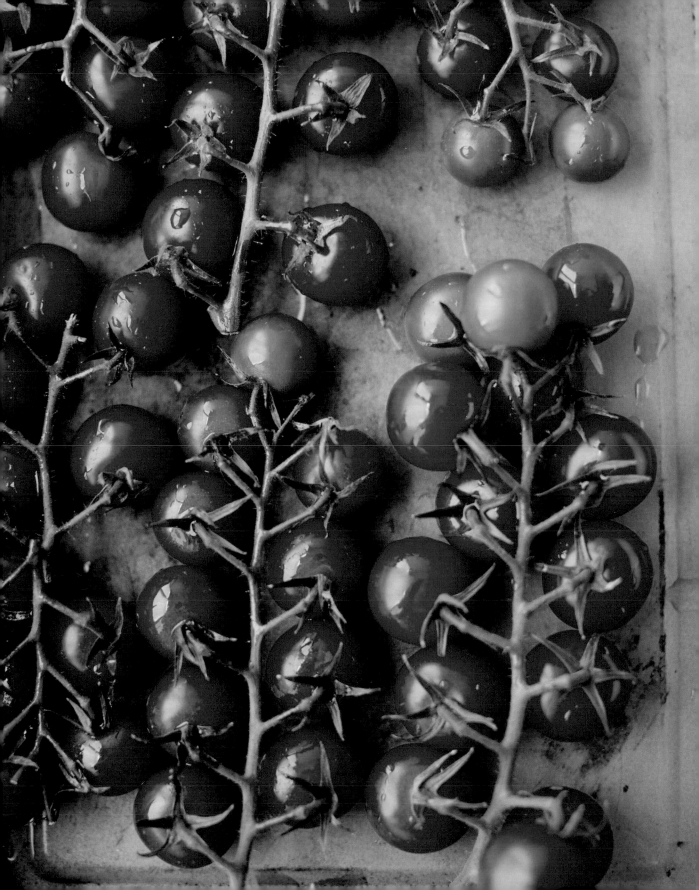

The savoury granola adds a nutritious, nutty crunch to this salad. It's worth making double the quantity to eat as a snack or perhaps sprinkle over yogurt for breakfast. If serving on sweet dishes, simply omit the tamari and store any leftover granola in an airtight container.

mixed leaves with savoury granola

150 g/5 oz. mixed salad
  leaves
2 nectarines, halved,
  stoned/pitted and
  sliced
125 g/4¼ oz. mozzarella,
  drained and torn
  into pieces
3 tablespoons extra
  virgin olive oil
freshly squeezed juice
  of ½ lemon
sea salt and freshly
  ground black pepper

SAVOURY GRANOLA
1 tablespoon buckwheat
  groats
1 tablespoon shelled
  hemp seeds
2 tablespoons sunflower
  seeds
2 tablespoons pumpkin
  seeds
a large handful of
  blanched almonds
1½ teaspoons tamari
  or light soy sauce
1½ teaspoons clear
  honey

Serves 4

To make the savoury granola, toast the buckwheat and hemp seeds in a large, dry frying pan/skillet over a medium heat for 2–3 minutes, tossing the pan regularly, until they start to smell toasted. Transfer to a bowl and add the sunflower and pumpkin seeds to the pan. Toast the seeds, again tossing the pan regularly, for 4–5 minutes, until starting to turn golden, then add to the bowl. Finally, add the almonds to the pan and toast for 5 minutes, turning occasionally, until starting to colour. Roughly chop the nuts and add to the bowl with the seeds.

Add the tamari and honey to the nuts and seeds and stir until combined, then leave to cool.

Meanwhile, place the salad leaves in a large serving dish and add the nectarines and mozzarella. Drizzle the olive oil and lemon juice over and season with salt and pepper. Gently toss the salad and sprinkle the granola over before serving.

SEEDS
Despite their diminutive size, seeds are particularly nutritious and add flavour and texture to all types of salads. Due to their high oil content, it's best to store them in an airtight container in the refrigerator.

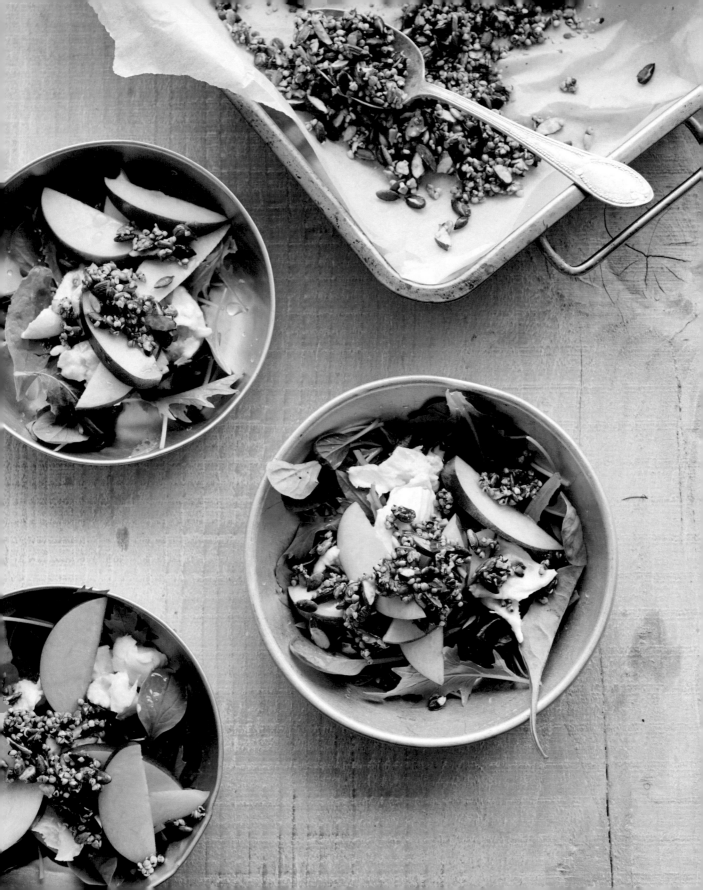

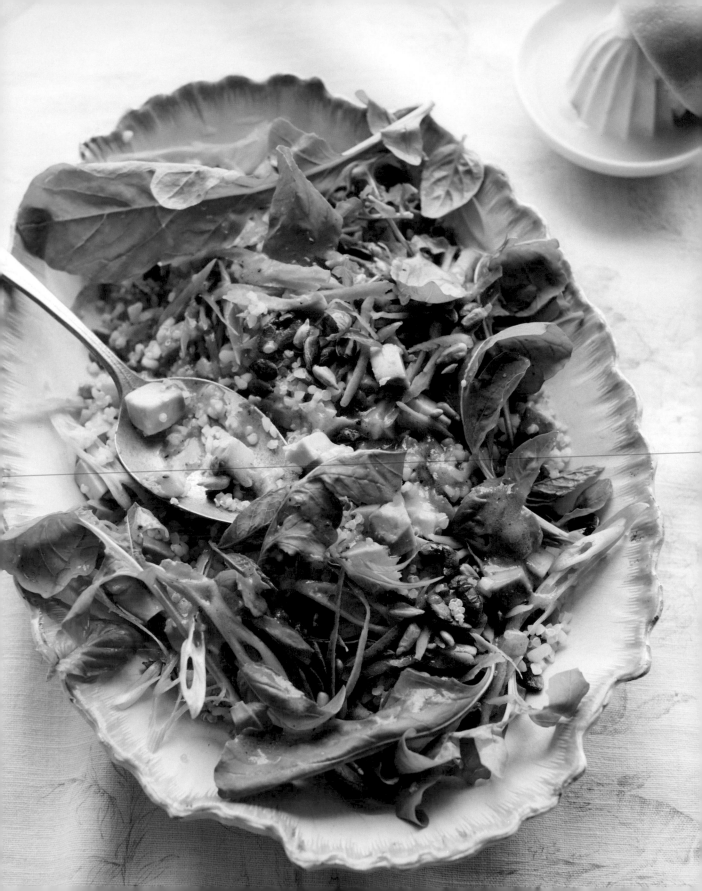

Packed with fresh, healthy ingredients, this makes a nutritious light meal or side dish. It is now possible to find bags of dried mixed grains, but you could save time by using ready-cooked grains.

mixed grain, avocado & toasted seed salad

150 g/5 oz. ready-mixed grains, such as quinoa and bulghur wheat
a squeeze of lemon juice
1 large avocado, halved, peeled, stoned/ pitted and cubed
100 g/3¾ oz. rocket/ arugula leaves
4 spring onions/ scallions, thinly sliced diagonally
1 carrot, coarsely grated
a large handful of basil leaves, freshly torn
6 tablespoons freshly chopped mint leaves

3 tablespoons sunflower seeds, toasted
2 tablespoons pumpkin seeds, toasted

DRESSING
5 tablespoons extra virgin olive oil
1 teaspoon clear honey
2 tablespoons white balsamic vinegar or white wine vinegar
1 teaspoon Dijon mustard
1 small garlic clove, finely chopped

Serves 4

Put the grains in a pan and cover with water. Bring to the boil, then turn the heat down and simmer, covered, for 15 minutes or until tender. Drain and set aside.

Meanwhile, squeeze a little lemon juice over the avocado to prevent it discolouring.

To make the dressing, whisk all the ingredients together in a bowl, season and set aside.

Put the rocket/arugula in a large serving bowl with the spring onions/scallions, carrot, herbs, avocado and cooked grains. Pour the dressing over and toss gently until combined. Sprinkle the seeds over before serving.

This warm salad is packed with robust flavours as well as wholesome ingredients. The kale is roasted in the oven and needs stirring into the salad just before serving so it stays crisp.

marinated mushroom, crispy kale & rice salad

100 g/½ cup brown basmati rice, rinsed
1 teaspoon ground turmeric
3 tablespoons dark soy sauce
2 tablespoons sweet chilli/chili sauce
300 g/11 oz. chestnut/ cremini mushrooms, sliced

175 g/6 oz. curly kale, tough stalks removed and leaves torn into large bite-sized pieces
2 teaspoons sesame oil
2 tablespoons coconut oil
2 handfuls of unsalted roasted cashews, roughly chopped
sea salt and freshly ground black pepper

Serves 4

Cook the rice following the packet instructions, stirring the turmeric into the cooking water. Drain, if necessary, and leave to stand, covered, for 10 minutes.

Meanwhile, mix together the soy sauce and sweet chilli/chili sauce in a bowl. Add the mushrooms and toss until coated in the marinade, then set aside.

Preheat the oven to 150°C (300°F) Gas 2. Toss the kale in the sesame oil and spread out on 1–2 baking sheets. Roast for 15 minutes, turning once, until crisp but not browned; keep an eye on it as it can easily burn.

Heat the coconut oil in a large frying pan/skillet over a medium-high heat and fry the mushrooms for 5 minutes. Pour off and retain any liquid from the mushrooms as this will form the dressing for the salad. Return the pan to the heat and cook the mushrooms for another 5 minutes, until they start to crisp.

Transfer the rice to a serving bowl and add the mushrooms and the cooking juices. Stir until combined and season, if necessary. Just before serving, stir in the crispy kale and sprinkle the cashews over.

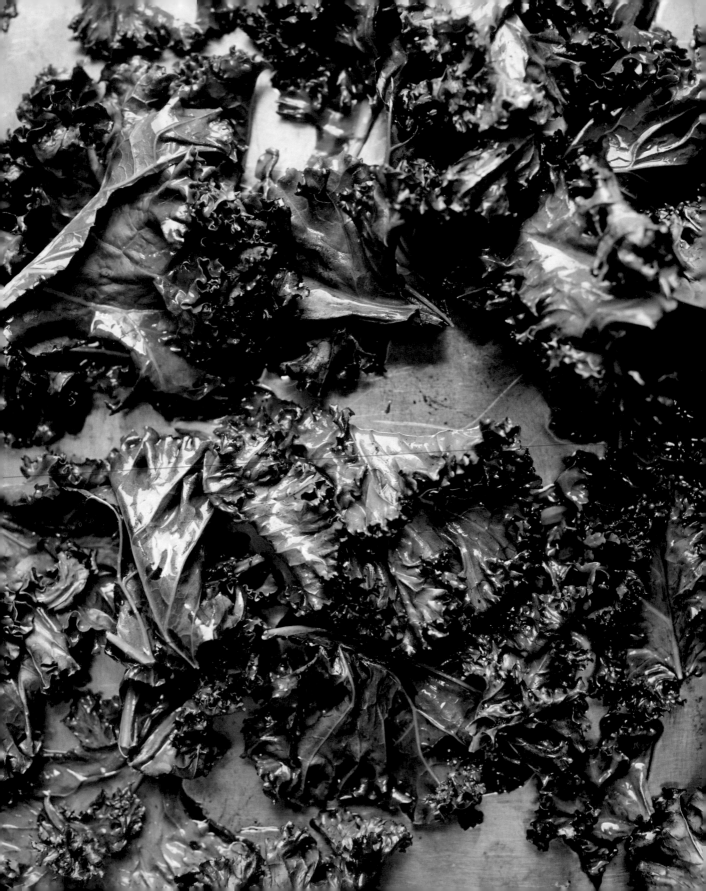

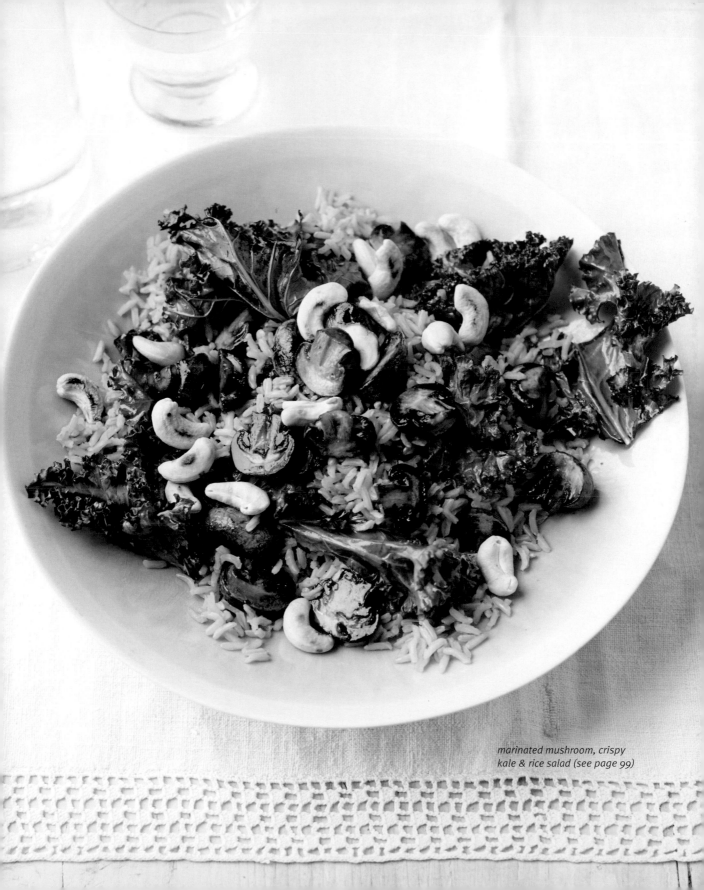

marinated mushroom, crispy
kale & rice salad (see page 99)

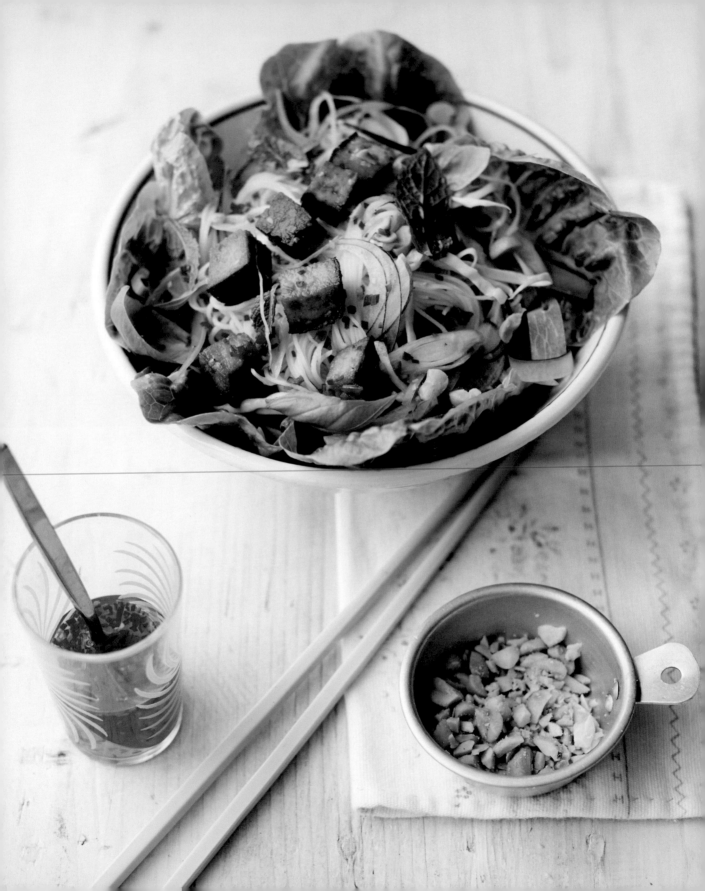

The ingredients for this Asian main meal salad may look on the long side, but it's very easy to prepare and can be made the night before if wanting to serve as a picnic lunch. If making in advance, assemble the salad just before serving.

rice noodle & smoked tofu salad

2 tablespoons coconut oil or sunflower oil

275 g/10 oz. smoked tofu, drained, patted dry, and cut into bite-sized cubes

200 g/7 oz. dried rice vermicelli noodles

1 carrot, halved crossways and thinly sliced into thin strips

10-cm/4-in. piece cucumber, quartered lengthways, seeded, and thinly sliced into strips

2 handfuls of shredded sweetheart/pointed cabbage

3 spring onions/ scallions, thinly sliced

½ red onion, finely sliced

2 handfuls of freshly chopped mint leaves

2 handfuls of freshly torn basil leaves

1 Little Gem/Bibb lettuce, leaves separated

75 g/⅓ cup salted peanuts, roughly chopped

DRESSING

5 tablespoons rice wine vinegar

4 teaspoons caster/ superfine sugar

1 tablespoon Thai fish sauce

1 red chilli/chile, seeded and diced

Serves 4

Heat the oil in a large frying pan/skillet over a medium heat and fry the tofu for 8–10 minutes, turning often, until golden and crisp. Drain on paper towels.

Meanwhile, prepare the noodles as instructed on the packet, then drain and refresh under cold running water and drain again. Transfer the noodles to a large bowl. Mix together all the ingredients for the dressing and pour over the noodles.

Add the carrot, cucumber, cabbage, spring onions/scallions, red onion and half the herbs to the noodles and toss until combined. Arrange the Little Gem/Bibb leaves on a large, flat serving plate and top with the noodle salad, smoked tofu, remaining herbs and peanuts.

SMOKED TOFU

The beauty of smoked tofu is that it doesn't need to be marinated before use. Try to find a brand that naturally smokes the tofu, rather than pump it with a smoke flavouring. Tofu is sold packed in water, so must be drained well and patted dry with paper towels before frying, otherwise you may have difficulty in getting it to crisp up.

Mostly used in soups and broths in Japan, soba noodles are also popular served cold in Asian-style salads. Made primarily from buckwheat, the thin noodles are coated in a light miso dressing.

soba noodles with miso dressing

200 g/7 oz. soba noodles or thin egg noodles
1 carrot, cut into thirds and finely shredded
1 red (bell) pepper, halved, seeded and finely shredded
4 spring onions/ scallions, finely shredded
50 g/2 oz. sugar snap peas, thinly sliced diagonally
a handful of radishes, thinly sliced
1 red chilli/chile, seeded and finely chopped
1-cm/½-in. piece fresh root ginger, peeled and finely chopped
4 teaspoons nori flakes (optional)
1 tablespoon sesame seeds, toasted

MISO DRESSING
3 tablespoons mirin
3 tablespoons tamari or light soy sauce
3 tablespoons sweet white miso paste

Serves 4

Cook the noodles in plenty of salted boiling water following the pack instructions, then drain and refresh under cold running water. Drain the noodles again, leaving them to drain while you prepare the rest of the ingredients.

Meanwhile, mix together all the ingredients for the dressing.

Put the carrot, red (bell) pepper, spring onions/ scallions, sugar snap peas, radishes, chilli/chile and ginger in a serving bowl. Add the cooked noodles and dressing and toss gently but thoroughly until combined. Sprinkle with the nori flakes, if using, and sesame seeds before serving.

MISO

Miso, a Japanese fermented paste made primarily from barley, soya beans or rice, imparts a rich, umami quality to dressings. Sweet white miso is mild is taste. Other varieties include yellow miso, which is slightly milder and sweeter in flavour than the more robust dark brown paste.

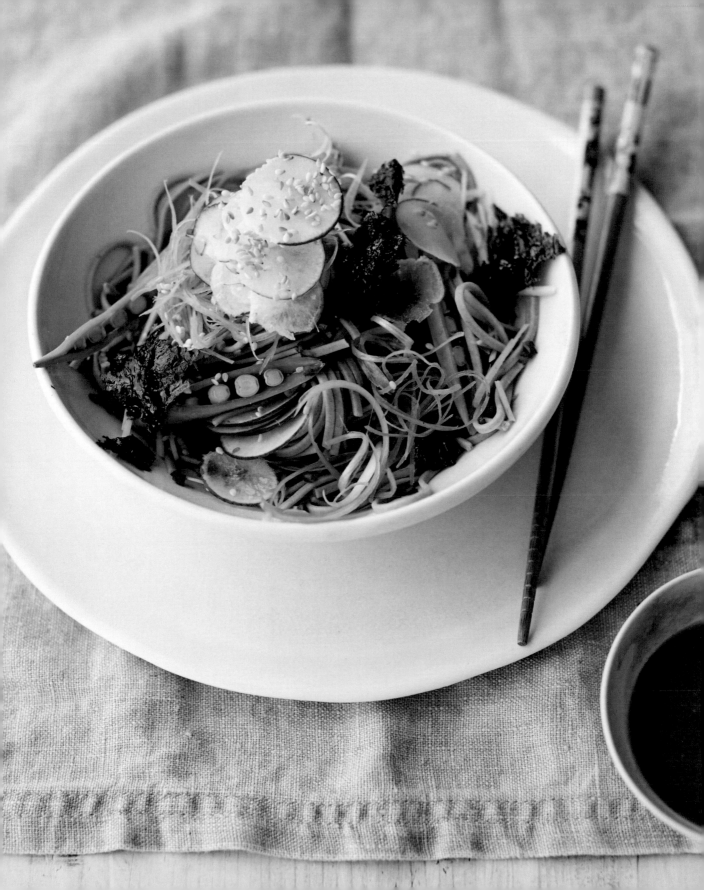

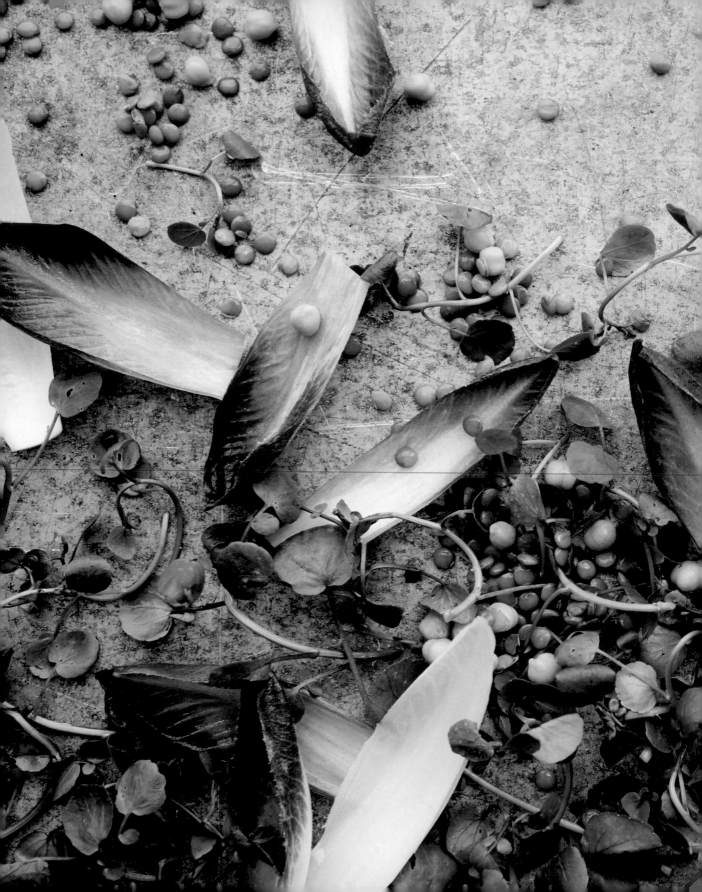

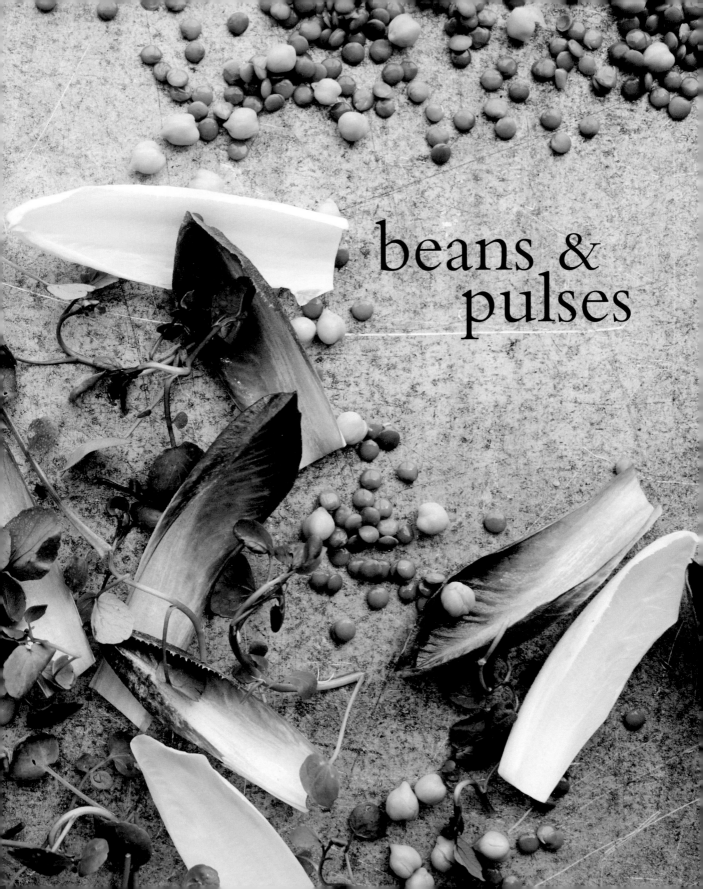

beans &
pulses

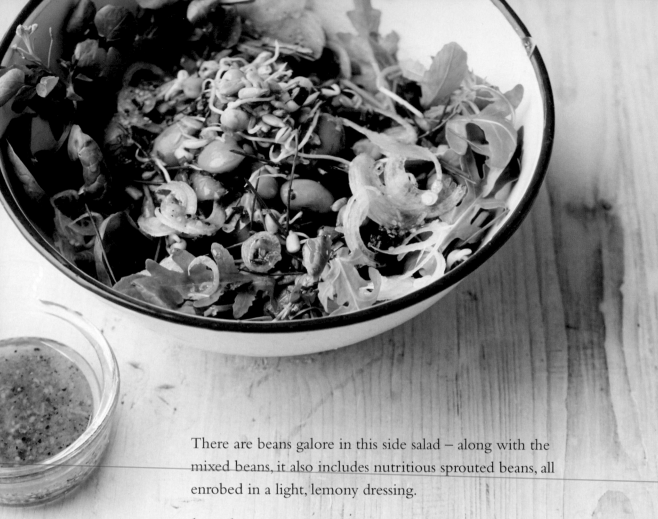

There are beans galore in this side salad – along with the mixed beans, it also includes nutritious sprouted beans, all enrobed in a light, lemony dressing.

herby mixed bean salad

400-g/14-oz. can mixed beans, drained and rinsed

125 g/4¼ oz. mixed rocket/arugula, watercress and spinach leaves

1 banana shallot, thinly sliced into rings

2 handfuls of mixed sprouted beans

3 tablespoons freshly chopped flat leaf parsley leaves

3 tablespoons freshly snipped chives

2 tablespoons sunflower seeds, toasted

DRESSING
4 tablespoons extra virgin olive oil
finely grated zest and freshly squeezed juice of ½ lemon
1 teaspoon wholegrain mustard
1 teaspoon clear honey
sea salt and freshly ground black pepper

Serves 4

Add all the ingredients for the dressing to a small jar, shake well until combined and season.

Put the mixed beans, salad leaves, shallot, sprouted beans and herbs in a serving bowl and spoon enough of the dressing over to coat. Toss until combined and garnish with the sunflower seeds before serving.

SPROUTED BEANS

Sprouting can boost the nutritional value of beans by up to a remarkable 60 per cent. Since they have a relatively short shelf life, it's best to buy in small quantities or perhaps sprout your own (see page 8–9).

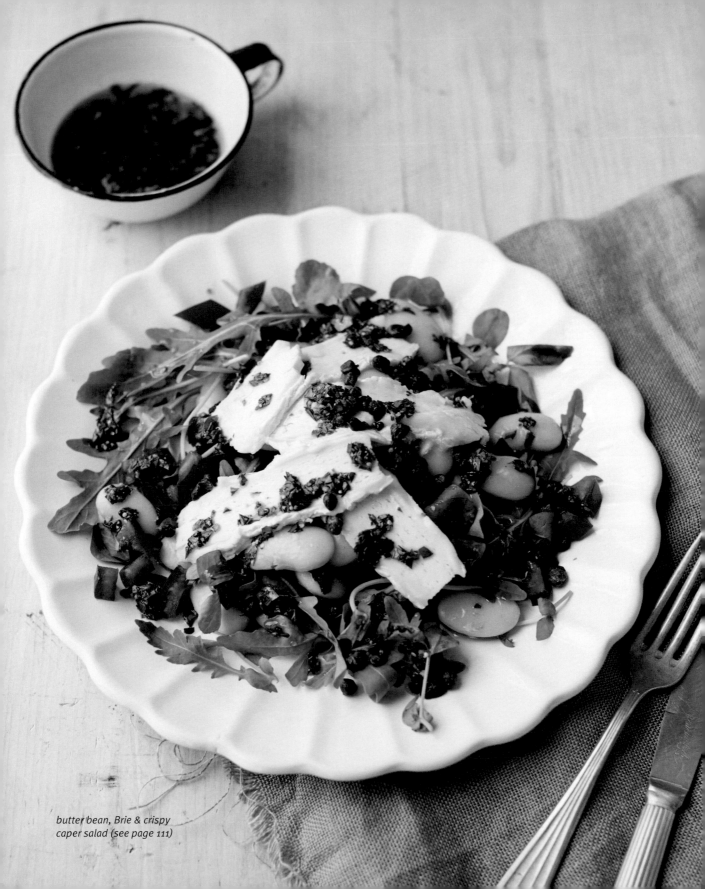

*butter bean, Brie & crispy
caper salad (see page 111)*

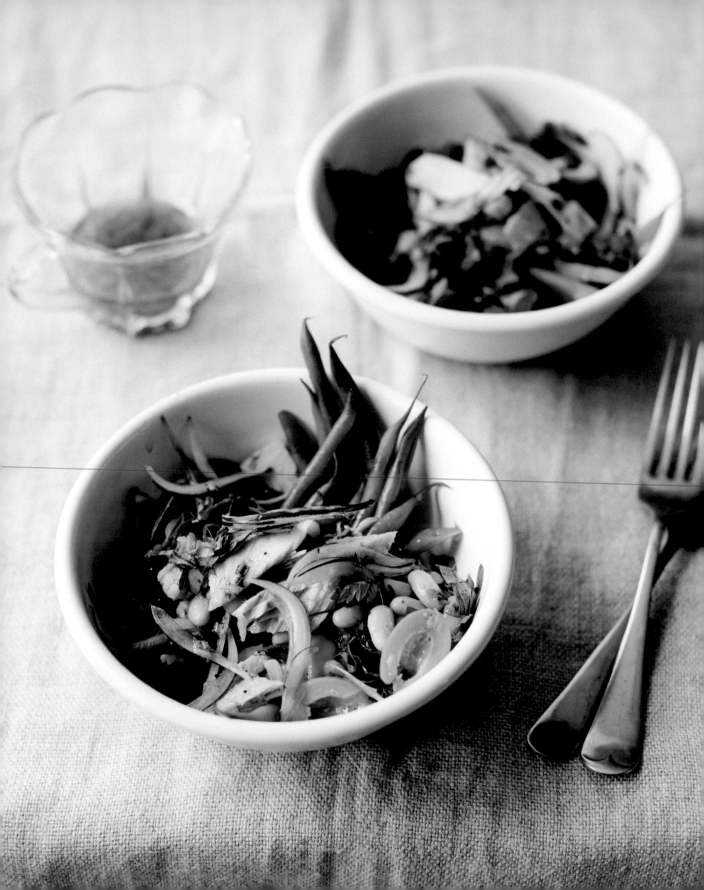

Often simple is best, and this recipe, which is loosely based on a salade Niçoise, is no exception. It makes a perfect light lunch served with crusty French bread, and you could also top it with a runny-yolked poached egg.

flageolet, tuna & olive salad

125 g/4¼ oz. fine green
   beans, trimmed
600 g/1 lb. 5 oz. canned
   flageolet/cannellini
   beans, drained and
   rinsed
200-g/7-oz. can tuna
   in olive oil, drained (oil
   reserved) and flaked
90 g/3½ oz. kalamata
   olives, drained
1 small red onion,
   thinly sliced

2 large handfuls of
   freshly chopped
   flat leaf parsley
a large handful of fresh
   oregano leaves

DRESSING
2 tablespoons extra
   virgin olive oil
1½ tablespoons red
   wine vinegar
1 small garlic clove,
   crushed
sea salt and freshly
   ground black pepper

Serves 4

Steam the green beans for 5 minutes or until tender, then refresh under cold running water.

Halve the green beans, then put them in a bowl with the flageolet/cannellini beans, tuna, olives, onion and herbs.

Mix together all the ingredients for the dressing, adding the oil from the drained tuna. Season and pour it over the salad. Toss gently until combined and serve at room temperature.

Crisp, salty and piquant, capers take on a new dimension when fried in olive oil; they certainly give this delicious bean salad a lift. The Brie is best when just ripe so it's soft and oozy without being too runny. Serve simply with crusty bread.

butter bean, Brie & crispy caper salad

6 tablespoons capers,
   drained, rinsed and
   patted dry
300 g/11 oz. drained
   canned butter/lima
   beans, rinsed
6 vine-ripened tomatoes,
   quartered, seeded
   and chopped
100 g/3¾ oz. rocket/
   arugula leaves
40 g/1½ oz. pea shoots
200 g/7 oz. just-ripe
   Brie, sliced

PARSLEY & GARLIC
DRESSING
5 tablespoons extra
   virgin olive oil, plus
   extra for frying
1 large garlic clove,
   peeled and halved
2 tablespoons white wine
   vinegar
1 teaspoon wholegrain
   mustard
4 tablespoons chopped
   flat leaf parsley
sea salt and freshly
   ground black pepper

Serves 4

Heat 1 tablespoon of the oil in a large frying pan/skillet over a medium heat and fry the capers for 3–5 minutes or until crisp and starting to colour; take care as they can splutter. Drain on paper towels and leave to cool.

Meanwhile, start to make the dressing. Gently heat the rest of the oil and the garlic in a small pan for 2 minutes. Take the pan off the heat and leave to infuse.

Tip the butter/lima beans into a large serving bowl and add the tomatoes, rocket/arugula and pea shoots.

Remove the garlic from the oil and pour it into a jug/pitcher. Whisk in the vinegar, mustard and parsley. Season, bearing in mind that the capers are salty, and pour the dressing over the salad. Toss to coat the salad in the dressing, and top with the Brie slices and capers.

With its lively flavours and vibrant colours, this salad makes a tasty light meal with warmed flatbreads. It features cooking chorizo sausages, but you could also use slices of ready-to-eat chorizo.

borlotti bean & avocado salad with chorizo

2 sweet potatoes,
   cut into wedges
200 g/7 oz. cooking
   chorizo sausages
2 x 400-g/14-oz. cans
   borlotti beans, drained
   and rinsed
1–2 green chillies/chiles,
   seeded and finely
   chopped, depending
   on taste
6 spring onions/scallions,
   finely chopped
1 large avocado, peeled,
   halved, stoned/pitted
   and cubed

3 handfuls of freshly
   chopped coriander/
   cilantro

DRESSING
5 tablespoons extra
   virgin olive oil
freshly squeezed juice
   of 1½ limes
½ teaspoon cumin
   seeds, toasted
sea salt and freshly
   ground black pepper

Serves 4

Preheat the oven to 190°C (375°F) Gas 5.

Toss the sweet potatoes in 1 tablespoon of the oil, season and transfer to a roasting pan. Spread out in an even layer and roast for 35–40 minutes, turning once, until tender and starting to colour.

Meanwhile, put the chorizo in a separate roasting pan and cook in the oven for 20 minutes, turning halfway, or until cooked. Leave the chorizo to cool slightly before slicing.

Mix together all the ingredients for the dressing and season. Put the borlotti beans in a serving bowl with the sweet potatoes, chillies/chiles, spring onions/scallions, avocado and coriander/cilantro. Add the chorizo and drizzle over enough of the dressing to coat, then toss until combined before serving.

The sweet-sour citrus dressing cuts through the rich saltiness of the bacon in this substantial salad. Look for apricots at the peak of ripeness for the best flavour, or choose flat ripe peaches instead.

haricot bean, lardon & apricot salad with citrus dressing

250 g/9 oz. bacon lardons
125 g/4¼ oz. baby
   spinach leaves
1 small red onion,
   cut into thin rings
600 g/1lb. 5 oz. canned
   haricot/navy beans,
   drained and rinsed
6 ripe apricots, halved,
   stoned/pitted and
   sliced
a bunch of radishes,
   sliced into rounds
a handful of basil leaves

CITRUS DRESSING
3 tablespoons extra
   virgin olive oil
1 teaspoon white
   balsamic vinegar
juice of ½ large orange
½ orange, peeled, pith
   removed and flesh
   chopped
1 red chilli/chile, seeded
   and diced
sea salt and freshly
   ground black pepper

Serves 4

Put the lardons in a large, dry frying pan/skillet over a medium heat and leave until the fat starts to run, then turn the heat up slightly and cook until crisp and golden, about 5 minutes. Drain on paper towels while you prepare the rest of the salad.

Meanwhile, to make the dressing, whisk together the olive oil, vinegar and orange juice in a bowl until combined. Stir in the orange flesh and chilli/chile and season.

Arrange the spinach leaves on a large serving plate. Top with the red onion, haricot/navy beans, apricots and radishes. Spoon the dressing over the top and garnish with the lardons and basil.

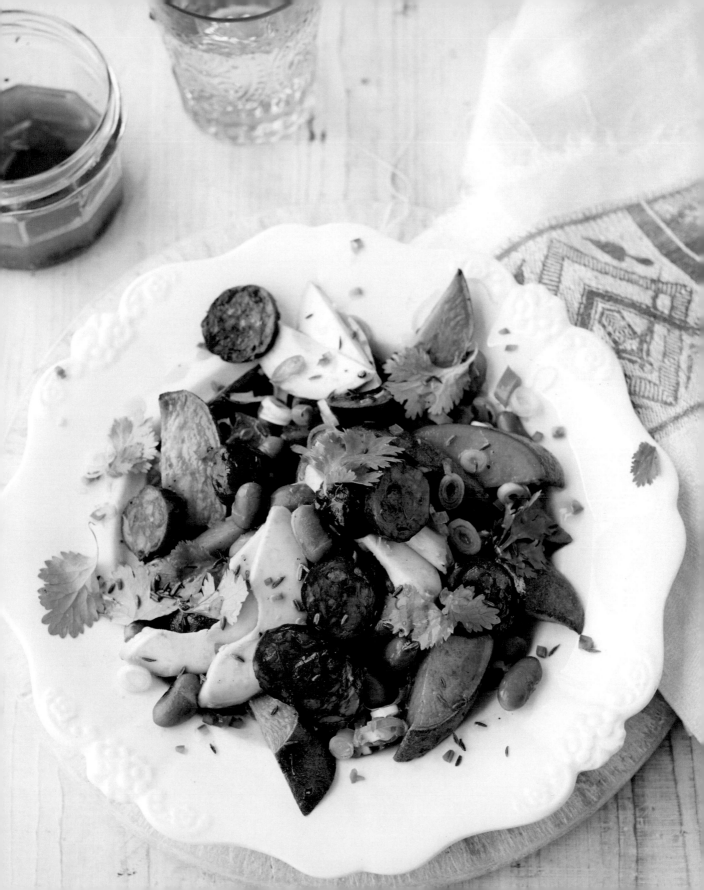

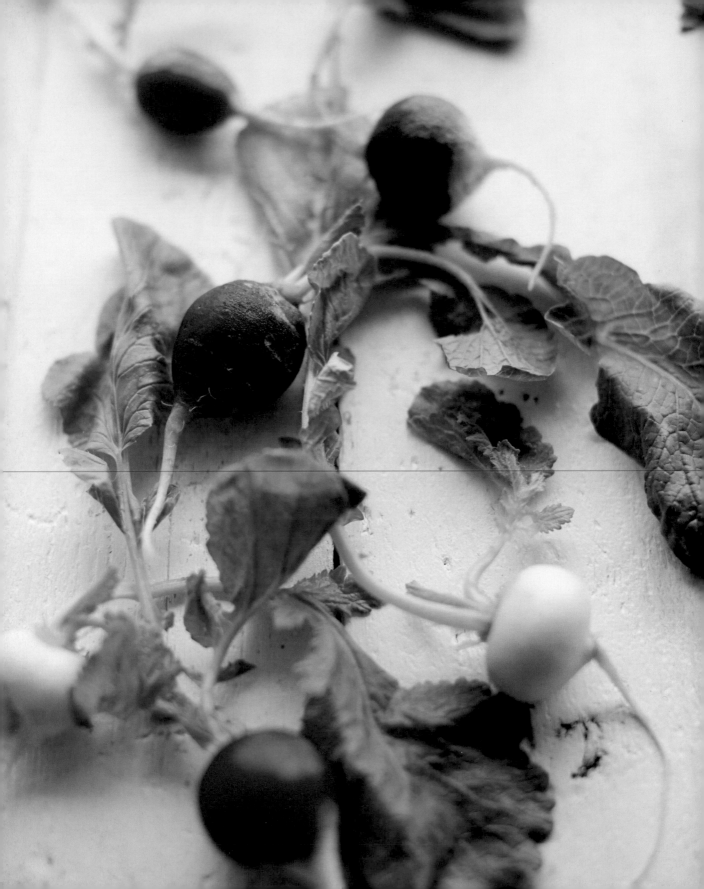

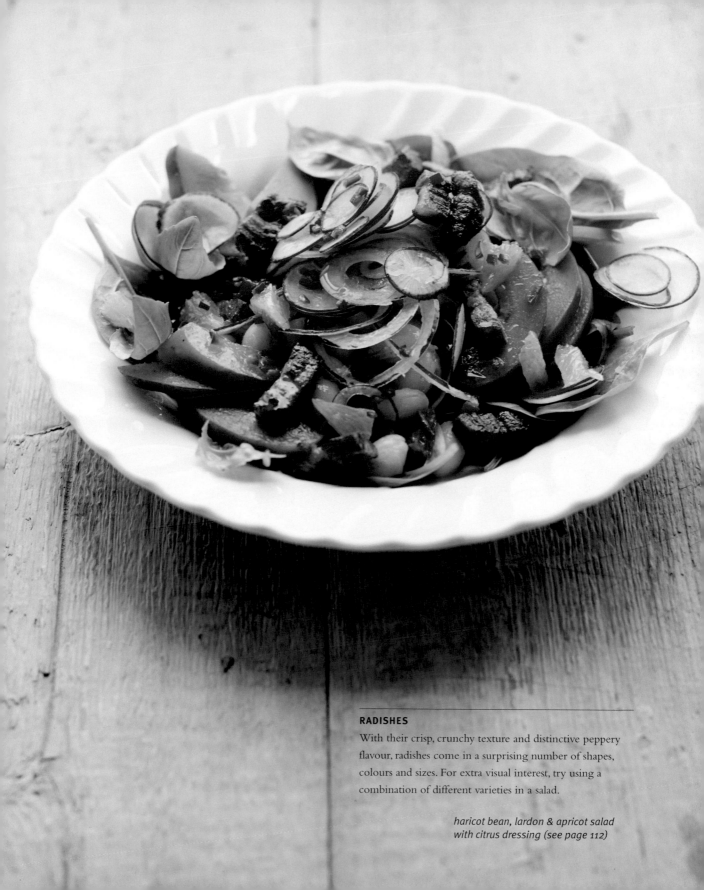

RADISHES

With their crisp, crunchy texture and distinctive peppery flavour, radishes come in a surprising number of shapes, colours and sizes. For extra visual interest, try using a combination of different varieties in a salad.

haricot bean, lardon & apricot salad
with citrus dressing (see page 112)

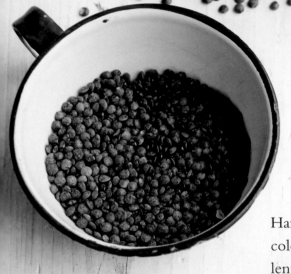

PUY LENTILS

The French Puy lentil with its dusky, blue-grey marbled skin is ideal for salads as it keeps its shape after cooking. Adding lentils to a salad is an easy way to add substance, turning it into a complete meal, especially when partnered with oily fish, lamb, poultry, eggs or cheese.

Harissa, the fiery North African spice paste, adds both colour and flavour to the dressing for this substantial Puy lentil salad. Oranges can be substituted for the grapefruit, if you prefer a slightly sweeter fruit. Serve with warm flatbreads on the side.

Puy lentils, grapefruit & feta cheese with harissa dressing

250 g/9 oz. dried Puy lentils

60 g/2 oz. watercress, tough stalks removed, separated into small sprigs

60 g/2 oz. baby spinach leaves, tough stalks trimmed

1 pink or red grapefruit, peeled, pith removed and segmented

1 small red onion, diced

a handful of mixed sprouted beans

200 g/7 oz. feta cheese, cubed

HARISSA DRESSING

5 tablespoons extra virgin olive oil

3 tablespoons freshly squeezed orange juice

1 teaspoon harissa paste

sea salt and freshly ground black pepper

Serves 4

Put the lentils in a pan and cover with plenty of water. Bring to the boil, then turn the heat down and simmer, part-covered, for 25 minutes or until tender. Drain and transfer the lentils to a serving bowl.

Meanwhile, mix together all the ingredients for the dressing, season and set aside.

Add the watercress and spinach to the serving bowl. Remove the membrane from the grapefruit segments over a dish and add the segments to the salad. Pour any juice from the grapefruit into the dressing.

Add the onion and mixed bean sprouts and pour the dressing over. Toss the salad until thoroughly combined and sprinkle the feta over before serving.

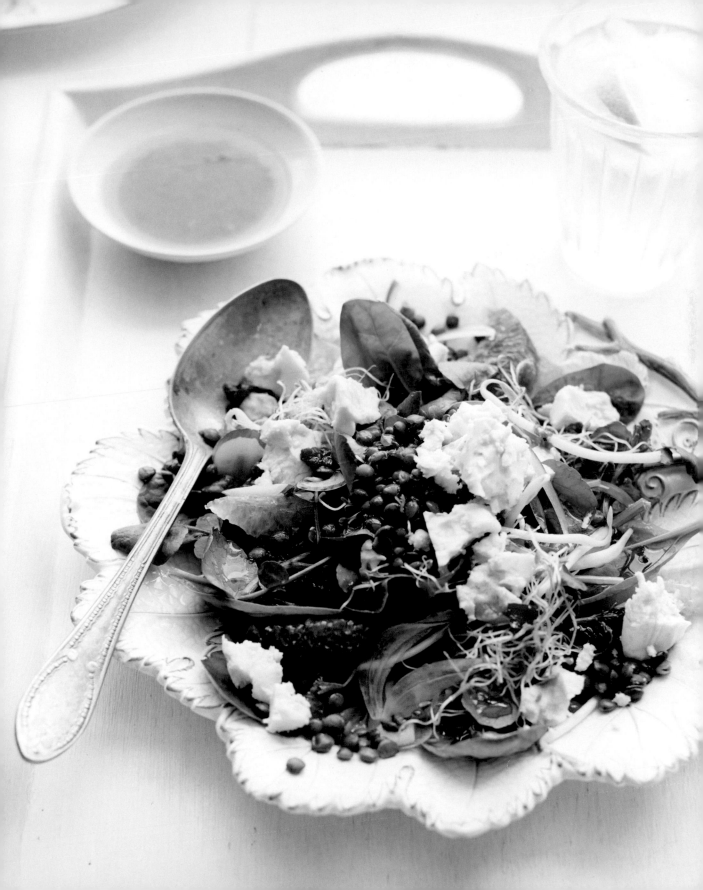

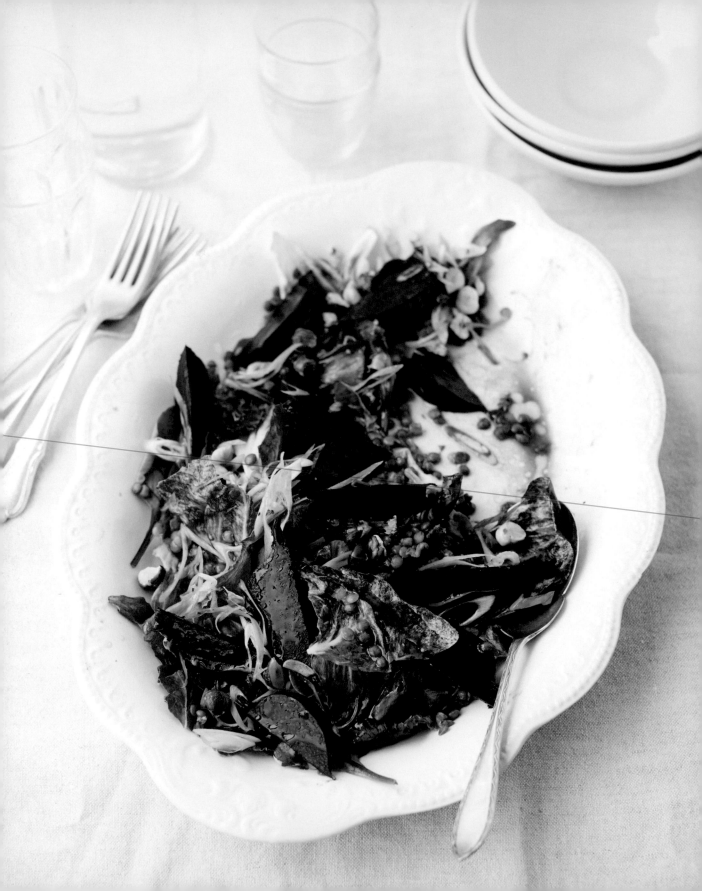

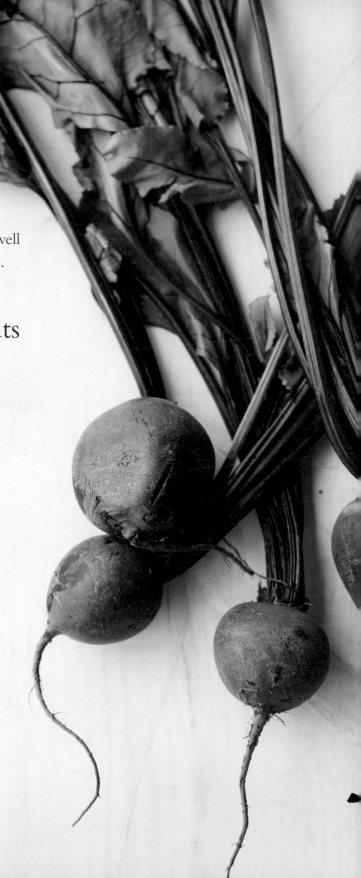

When buying raspberry vinegar opt for quality, if you can. The best ones are slightly syrupy in texture, with a fragrant natural hint of raspberries that just lifts a salad to new heights and works particularly well with the beetroot/beets, lentils and hazelnuts.

green lentil, red leaf & beetroot with hazelnuts

150 g/5 oz. dried
  green lentils
125 g/4¼ oz. mixed
  red salad leaves
1 radicchio, leaves
  separated and halved
  crossways, if large
200 g/7 oz. cooked
  beetroot/beets
  in natural juice,
  drained and cubed
2 spring onions/
  scallions, finely sliced
3 tablespoons freshly
  chopped flat leaf
  parsley

60 g/½ cup hazelnuts,
  toasted and halved

RASPBERRY DRESSING
4 tablespoons extra
  virgin olive oil
2 tablespoons
  good-quality
  raspberry vinegar
1 heaped teaspoon
  clear honey
1 teaspoon Dijon mustard
sea salt and freshly
  ground black pepper

Serves 4

Put the lentils in a pan and cover generously with water. Bring to the boil, then turn the heat down and simmer, part-covered, for 25 minutes or until tender. Drain the lentils and set aside.

Meanwhile, make the raspberry dressing. Put all the ingredients in a screw-top jar and shake until combined, then season.

Arrange the salad leaves and radicchio on a large serving plate and top with the lentils, beetroot/beets and spring onions/scallions. Spoon the dressing over, toss lightly to combine, then top with the parsley and hazelnuts before serving.

Chimichurri, the feisty Argentinian version of pesto, makes a great base for a salad dressing. You'll have some left over so just keep it in a jar in the fridge for up to 2 weeks. It's great poured over pasta, noodles, rice or beans, as here.

black bean, roasted pepper & chimichurri dressing

2 red-fleshed sweet potatoes, peeled and cut into bite-sized cubes

2 red (bell) peppers, quartered and seeded

100 g/3¾ oz. rocket/arugula leaves

400 g/14 oz. canned black beans, drained and rinsed

4 tablespoons pumpkin seeds, toasted

CHIMICHURRI DRESSING

15 g/½ oz. flat leaf parsley leaves, finely chopped

8 g/¼ oz. oregano leaves, finely chopped

1 large garlic clove, crushed

freshly squeezed juice of ½ lemon

1 red chilli/chile, seeded and finely chopped

6 tablespoons extra virgin olive oil, plus extra for brushing

sea salt and freshly ground black pepper

Serves 4

Preheat the oven to 200°C (400°F) Gas 6.

Brush the sweet potatoes with olive oil and roast in a roasting pan in the preheated oven for 35–40 minutes, turning once, until tender.

Meanwhile, brush both sides of the red (bell) peppers with olive oil and arrange on a baking sheet. Roast for 35 minutes, turning once, or until tender and blackened in places. Put the peppers in a bowl and cover with clingfilm/plastic wrap; this will make them easier to peel.

While the sweet potatoes and (bell) peppers are roasting, make the chimichurri dressing. Put the parsley, oregano, garlic, lemon juice, chilli/chile and olive oil in a food processor or blender, season, and process until coarsely chopped. (The mixture can also be chopped by hand.) Set aside.

Peel off the skin of the (bell) peppers and cut into bite-sized pieces. Arrange the rocket/arugula leaves on 4 serving plates and top with the sweet potatoes, black beans and red (bell) pepper. Spoon enough of the dressing over the salad to lightly coat it and sprinkle the pumpkin seeds on top before serving.

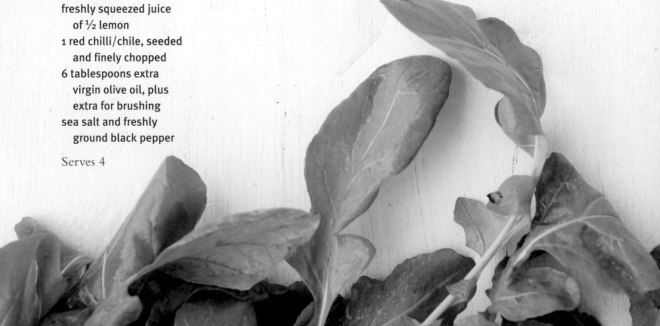

PUMPKIN SEEDS

Toasting gives nutritious pumpkin seeds a lovely nutty flavour and crunchy texture. Small quantities of seeds can be toasted in a large, dry frying pan/skillet, tossing them occasionally until they start to colour, but take care as they can pop out of or splutter in the pan as they heat up.

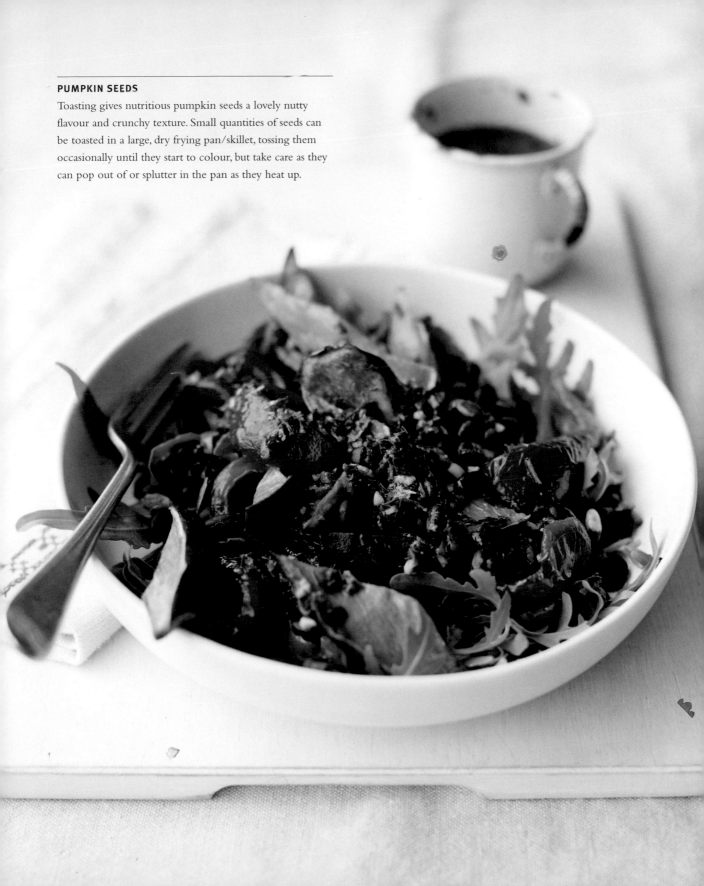

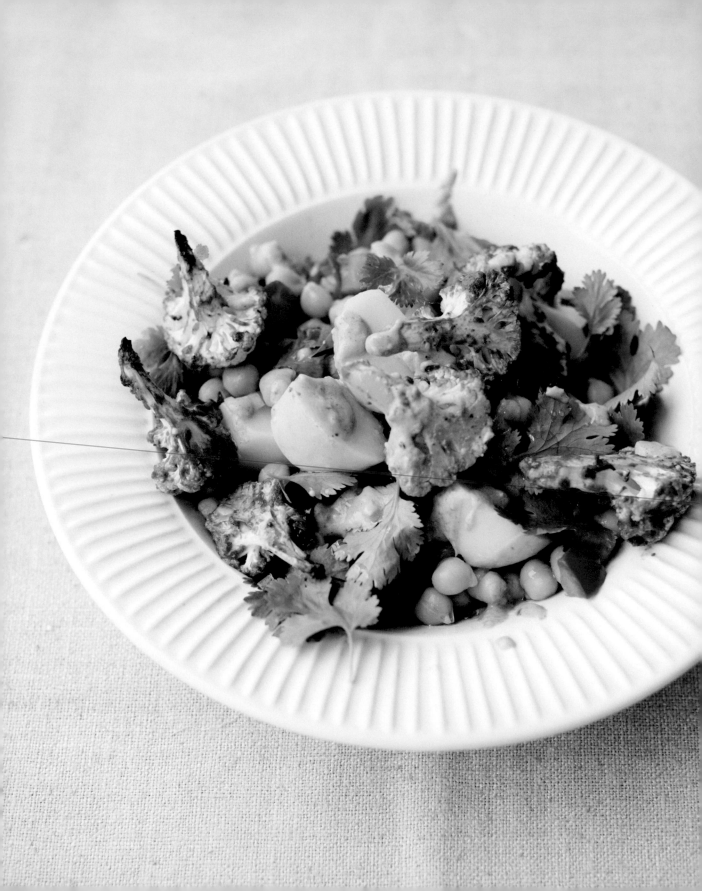

Cauliflower takes on a new lease of life when marinated in spices and roasted until just tender. Here, it is served on top of an Indian-inspired chickpea, tomato and potato salad with a tangy tamarind and yogurt dressing.

chickpea & spiced cauliflower salad with tamarind dressing

3 tablespoons cold-pressed rapeseed oil or light olive oil
2 teaspoons ground turmeric
2 tablespoons tikka curry paste
freshly squeezed juice of ½ lime
1 cauliflower, cut into florets, stalks trimmed
400 g/14 oz. new potatoes, halved
400 g/14 oz. canned chickpeas, drained and rinsed
1 small red onion, diced
4 tomatoes, seeded and diced

2 large handfuls of freshly chopped coriander/cilantro leaves
sea salt and freshly ground black pepper

TAMARIND DRESSING
3 tablespoons tamarind paste
2.5-cm/1-in. piece fresh root ginger, peeled and diced
freshly squeezed juice of ½ lime
6 tablespoons natural/plain yogurt

Serves 4

Preheat the oven to 200°C (400°F) Gas 6.

Mix together the oil, turmeric, curry paste and lime juice in a shallow bowl, then season. Add the cauliflower and turn to coat in the paste. Transfer to a roasting pan and roast for 10–15 minutes, depending on the size of the florets, turning once, until tender.

Meanwhile, cook the potatoes in a pan of boiling water for 12–15 minutes, until tender. Drain and leave until cool enough to handle, then peel off the skins and cut into cubes.

Mix together all the ingredients for the dressing, and season with salt and pepper.

Put the potatoes in a serving bowl with the chickpeas, onion, tomatoes and half the coriander/cilantro. Spoon the dressing over and mix gently until combined. Top with the roasted cauliflower and the remaining coriander/cilantro.

TAMARIND

In its natural state, tamarind fruit looks like a long brown pod, inside of which is a sticky, tangy, seedy pulp. It's more commonly sold as a paste or in a block – with or without seeds – and adds a sweet-sour note to dishes.

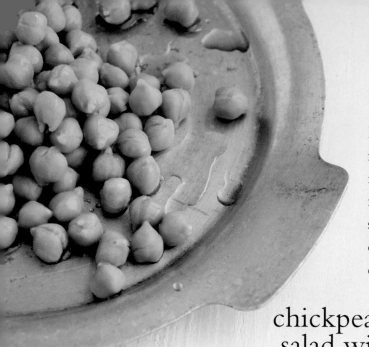

I pretty much always have a pot of dukkah in the refrigerator. This fragrant Egyptian mix of spices, nuts, seeds and dried chilli flakes/hot pepper flakes is delicious sprinkled over salads or roasted vegetables, or stirred into olive oil to make a quick and easy dip to serve with warm pitta bread.

chickpea, squash & spinach salad with dukkah

1 teaspoon smoked hot paprika

1 tablespoon extra virgin olive oil

400 g/14 oz. butternut squash, peeled, seeded and sliced into wedges

150 g/5 oz. baby spinach leaves, tough stalks trimmed

2 avocados, peeled, halved, stoned/pitted and cubed

400 g/14 oz. canned chickpeas, drained and rinsed

1 small red onion, diced

a large handful of coriander/cilantro leaves

2 tablespoons dukkah (see page 11)

LEMON AND CORIANDER DRESSING

1 teaspoon coriander seeds

5 tablespoons extra virgin olive oil

finely grated zest and freshly squeezed juice of 1 small lemon

sea salt and freshly ground black pepper

Serves 4

Preheat the oven to 200°C (400°F) Gas 6.

Mix the paprika with the oil in a large bowl, season, stir in the squash and turn until evenly coated. Roast the squash in the preheated oven for 30–35 minutes, turning once, until tender and golden.

Meanwhile, to make the dressing, put the coriander seeds in a large, dry frying pan/skillet and toast for 2–3 minutes, shaking the pan occasionally, until they smell aromatic and start to colour. Grind using a pestle and mortar to a coarse powder. Transfer the ground coriander seeds to a bowl and mix in the oil and lemon zest and juice. Season and set aside.

Put the spinach in a large serving bowl and add the roasted squash, avocados, chickpeas, red onion and half the fresh coriander/cilantro. Pour enough of the dressing over to coat and turn gently until combined.

Just before serving, sprinkle the dukkah and the remaining fresh coriander/cilantro over.

CHICKPEAS

Chickpeas, or garbanzo beans, are a popular feature of Middle Eastern, Indian, Mediterranean and North African dishes, as in this salad. They add a nutty bite and valuable amounts of protein.

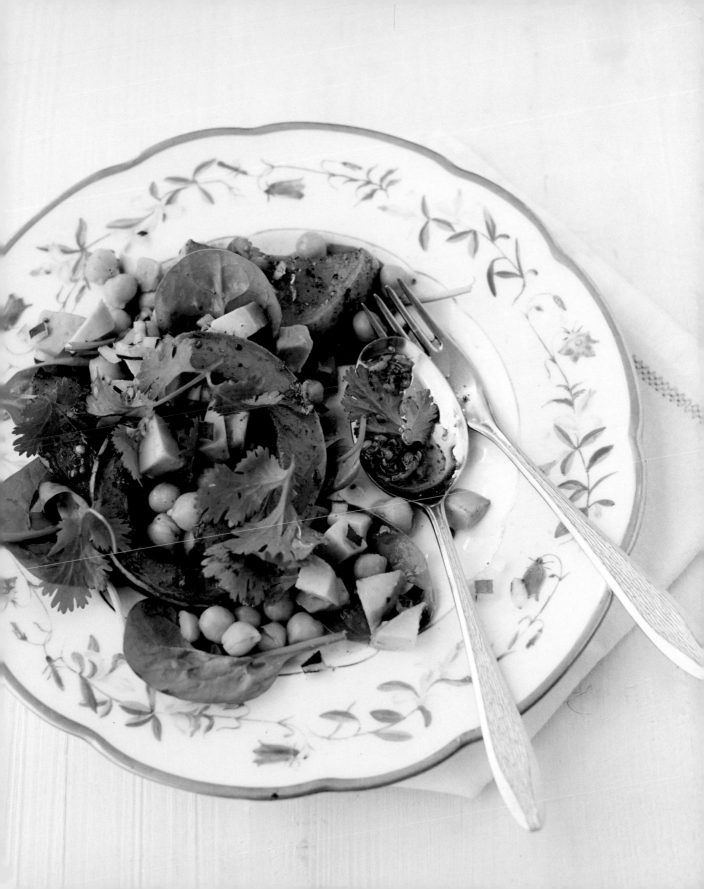

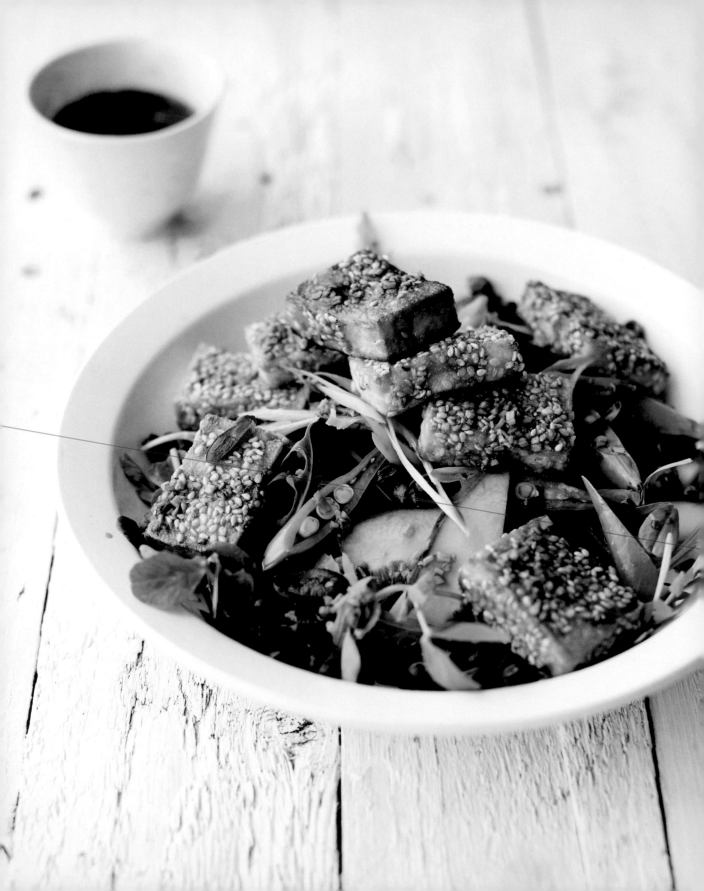

In this Asian-inspired salad, the sesame seeds form a thick, nutty crust around slices of tamari-marinated tofu, which are then served on top of an aduki bean and pea shoot salad.

sesame-coated tofu with aduki bean salad

450 g/1 lb. tofu, drained, patted dry and sliced into 8 slices about 1 cm/½ in. thick

2 tablespoons tamari or light soy sauce

4 heaped teaspoons cornflour/cornstarch

6 heaped tablespoons sesame seeds

125 g/4¼ oz. canned aduki beans, drained and rinsed

11-cm/4-in piece cucumber, quartered lengthways and thinly sliced

3 spring onions/ scallions, thinly sliced diagonally

120 g/4 oz. pea shoots and mixed leaves

2 handfuls of sugar snap peas, sliced diagonally

1 red chilli/chile, seeded and thinly sliced

sunflower oil, for frying

DRESSING

2 tablespoons tamari or light soy sauce

2 tablespoons freshly squeezed lime juice

1 teaspoon caster/ superfine sugar

1-cm/½-in. piece fresh root ginger, peeled and finely chopped

Serves 4

Put the tofu in a shallow dish and pour the tamari over. Turn the tofu to coat it in the tamari and leave to marinate for 1 hour, spooning the tamari over the tofu occasionally.

Mix together the cornflour/cornstarch and sesame seeds in a second shallow dish. Add the tofu in batches and turn until evenly coated in the mixture. Pour enough sunflower oil into a large frying pan/skillet to shallow-fry the tofu. Fry the tofu over a medium heat in two batches for 2–3 minutes on each side until golden, then drain on paper towels.

Meanwhile, mix together all the ingredients for the dressing and stir to dissolve the sugar.

Put the aduki beans, cucumber, two of the spring onions/scallions, the pea shoots and mixed leaves, sugar snap peas and half the chilli/chile in a large serving dish. Pour enough of the dressing over to coat and toss gently until combined.

Pile the sesame-coated tofu on top of the salad and sprinkle over the remaining spring onions/scallions and chilli/chile.

TOFU

Made from cooked soya beans, tofu (also called bean curd) responds well to being combined with strong flavours. Its naturally mild taste and soft texture combine beautifully with crisp, raw vegetables and punchy dressings.

This takes many of the features of the classic Tuscan panzanella salad and adapts them by adding a chipotle-infused dressing, red kidney beans and plenty of fresh herbs.

Mexican panzanella

2 large corn-on-the-cobs,
  leaves discarded
2 soft corn tortillas
350 g/12 oz. canned
  drained red kidney
  beans, rinsed
1 large red (bell) pepper,
  seeded and cut into
  bite-sized pieces
1 small red onion,
  roughly chopped
6 tomatoes, seeded and
  roughly chopped
100 g/3¾ oz. radishes,
  sliced into rounds
1 large avocado, peeled,
  halved, stoned/pitted
  and cubed
2 handfuls of freshly
  chopped coriander/
  cilantro
2 handfuls of freshly
  chopped flat-leaf
  parsley

DRESSING
1 dried chipotle chilli/
  chile or 1–2 teaspoons
  chipotle paste, to taste
4 tablespoons extra
  virgin olive oil, plus
  extra for brushing
freshly squeezed juice
  of 1½ limes
1 teaspoon ground cumin
½ teaspoon dried
  oregano
sea salt and freshly
  ground black pepper

Serves 4

To start the dressing, cover the dried chipotle chilli/chile with just-boiled water in a small bowl and leave for 15 minutes to soften. Drain, cut the chilli/chile open and discard the seeds, then finely chop the flesh.

Meanwhile, put the corn cobs in a pan, cover with water and bring to the boil, then turn the heat down and simmer, part-covered, for 12 minutes or until tender. Drain and refresh under cold running water, then drain again. Carefully slice the kernels off the cob and put them in a serving bowl.

While the corn is cooking, lightly coat a frying pan/skillet with oil and toast the tortillas, one at a time, for 3 minutes, turning once, until golden and crisp; they will crisp up further when cooled. Let cool.

Finish making the dressing by combining the chopped chipotle, olive oil, lime juice, cumin and oregano, then season.

Add the kidney beans, red (bell) pepper, onion, tomatoes, radishes, avocado and herbs to the serving bowl. Spoon enough of the dressing over to coat and toss gently until combined. Break the corn tortillas into pieces and add to the salad just before serving.

CHIPOTLE CHILLI/CHILE
This Mexican, smoke-dried jalapeño chilli/chile adds a delicious warm, smoky heat to dressings, sauces and stews.

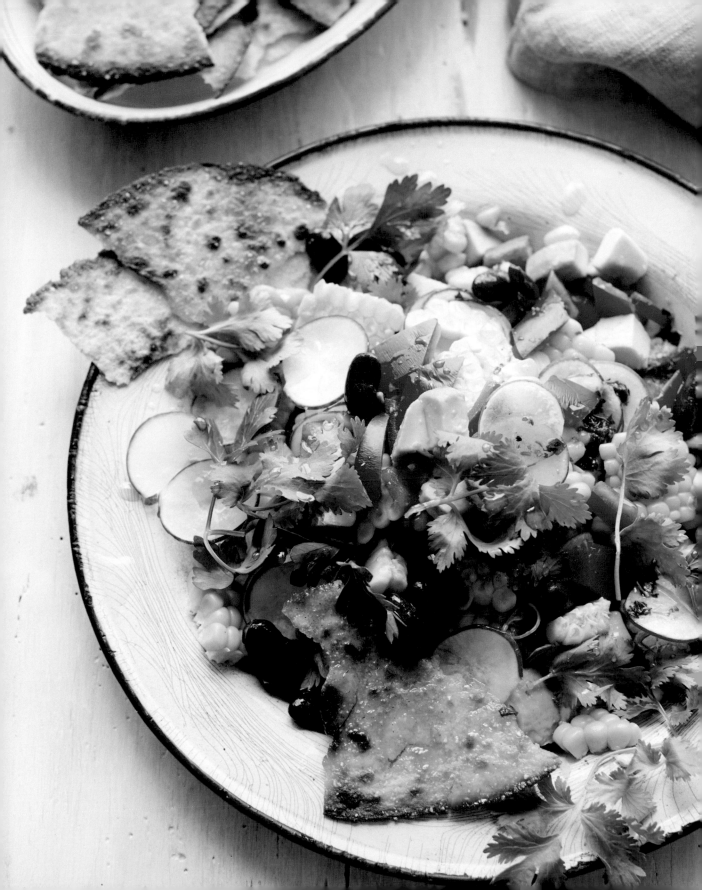

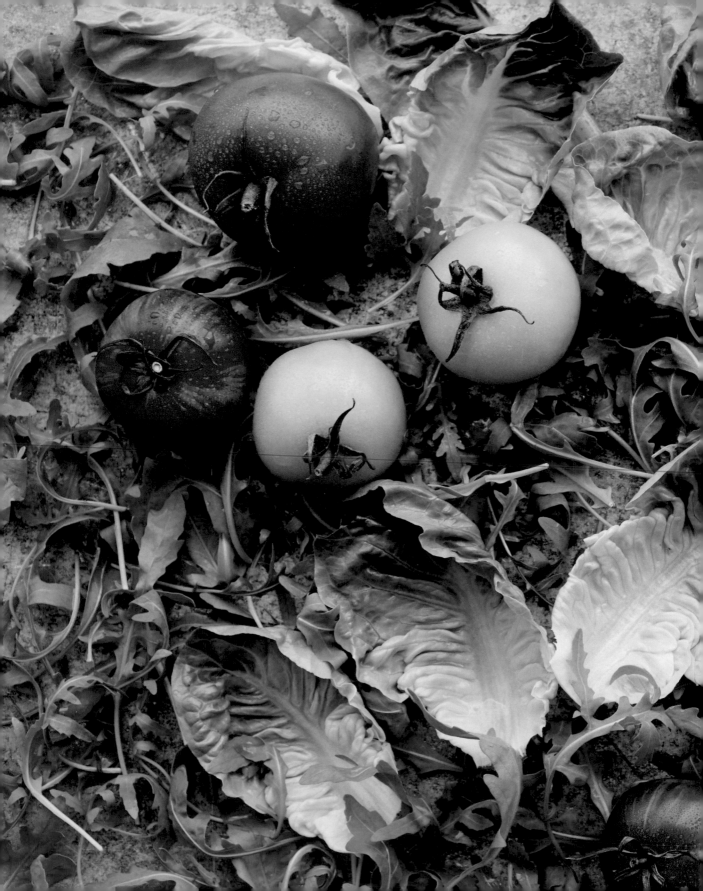

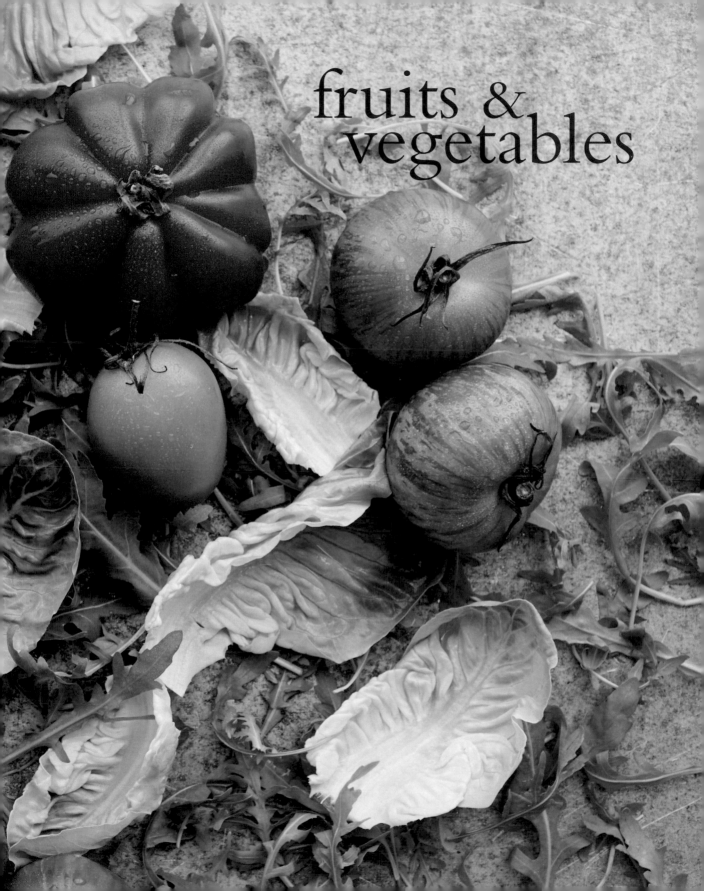

fruits &
vegetables

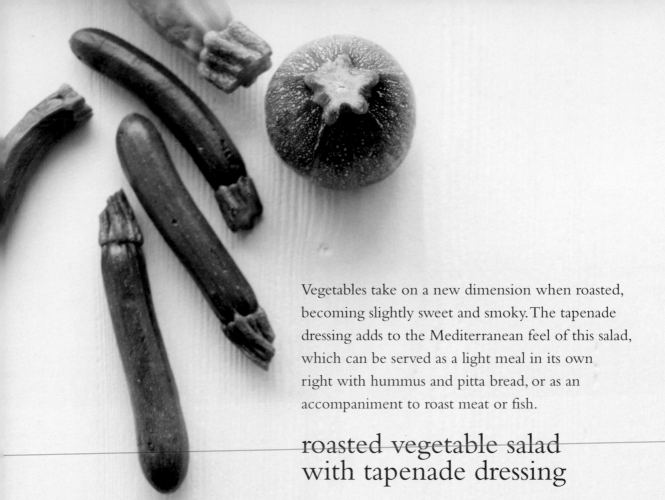

Vegetables take on a new dimension when roasted, becoming slightly sweet and smoky. The tapenade dressing adds to the Mediterranean feel of this salad, which can be served as a light meal in its own right with hummus and pitta bread, or as an accompaniment to roast meat or fish.

roasted vegetable salad with tapenade dressing

2 tablespoons extra virgin olive oil

2 tablespoons balsamic vinegar

8 baby courgettes/zucchini, halved lengthways

2 onions, halved and each half cut into 3 wedges

1 large red (bell) pepper, halved, seeded and cut into long wedges

1 large orange (bell) pepper, halved, seeded and cut into long wedges

2 fennel bulbs, cut into wedges

TAPENADE DRESSING

60 g/2½ oz. pitted black olives, drained

1 tablespoon capers, rinsed and patted dry

1 garlic clove, crushed

5 tablespoons extra virgin olive oil

a large handful of flat leaf parsley leaves

sea salt and freshly ground black pepper

Serves 4

Mix the olive oil and balsamic vinegar together in a large, shallow dish. Add the prepared vegetables, turn to coat them in the marinade, then leave to marinate while the oven is heating.

Preheat the oven to 200°C (400°F) Gas 6.

Turn out the vegetables into 2 large roasting pans and spread out into an even layer. Roast for 20 minutes, remove the courgettes/zucchini if tender, then return the rest of the vegetables to the oven and cook for a further 20 minutes, or until tender and blackened in places.

Meanwhile, to make the tapenade dressing, put the olives in a food processor or blender with the capers, garlic, olive oil and parsley, then pulse briefly until finely chopped and season to taste. Alternatively, coarsely chop all the ingredients by hand.

Serve the roasted vegetables warm or at room temperature, with some of the tapenade spooned over the top. (Transfer any remaining dressing to an airtight container and store in the refrigerator for up to 1 week.)

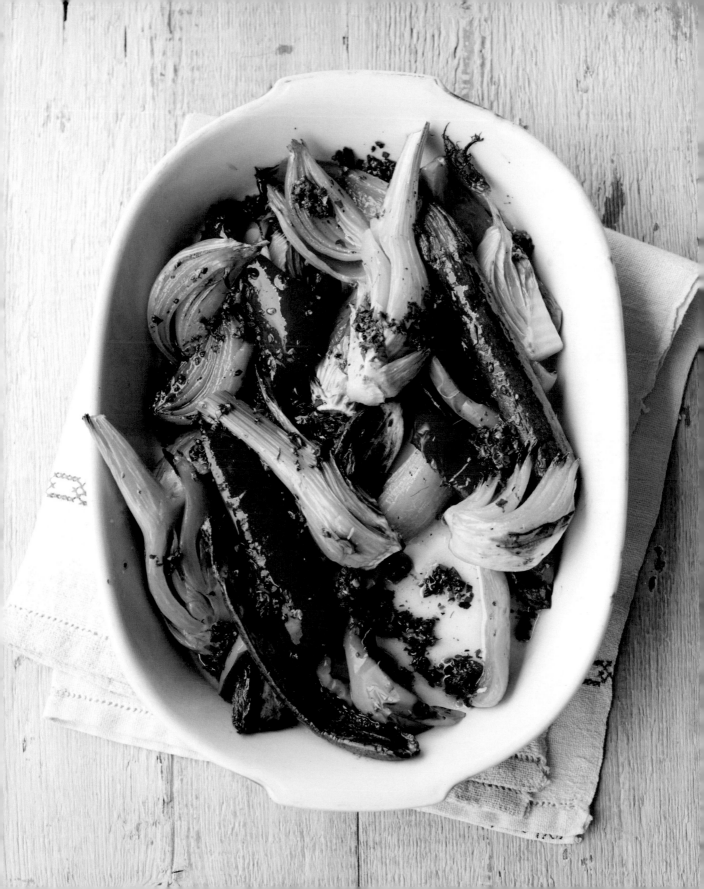

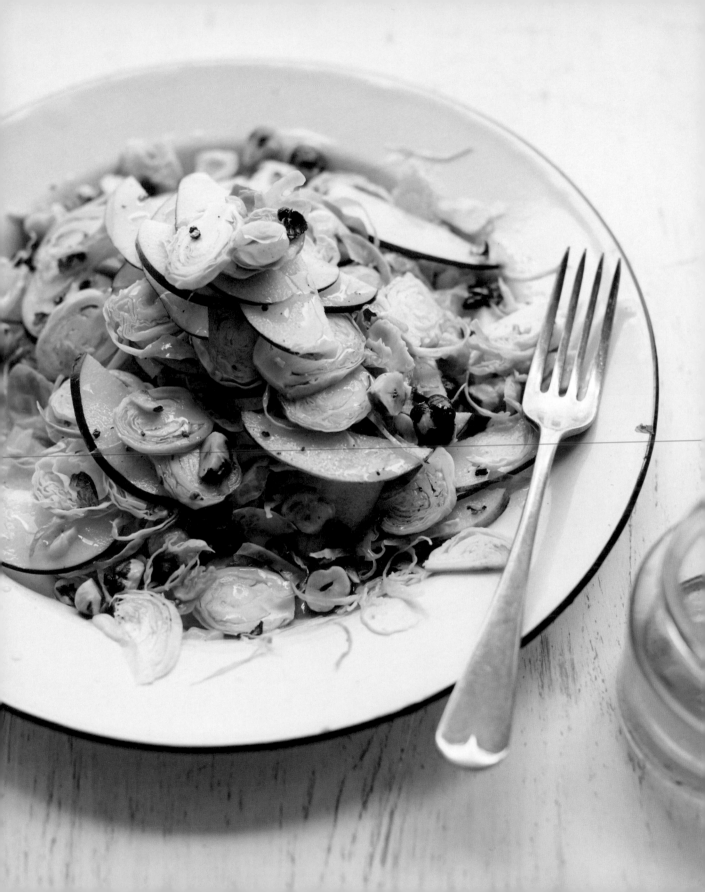

If the appeal of Brussels sprouts is blighted by the memory of over-cooked ones served at Christmas, this salad could win you over. Sprouts take on a new lease of life when served raw with toasted hazelnuts and apple.

Brussels sprout & apple salad with toasted hazelnuts

300 g/11 oz. Brussels
  sprouts, tough outer
  leaves removed
1 crisp, red-skinned
  eating apple, quartered,
  cored and sliced
squeeze of lemon juice
50 g/½ cup hazelnuts,
  toasted (see page 11)
  and roughly chopped

DRESSING
2 tablespoons
  hazelnut oil
2 tablespoons olive oil
1 tablespoon apple
  cider vinegar
sea salt and freshly
  ground black pepper

Serves 4

Cut the sprouts into thin slices using a mandoline and put into a serving bowl.

Toss the apple slices in a little lemon juice to prevent them discolouring, then add to the sprouts.

Mix together all the ingredients for the dressing, season and pour it over the salad. Toss until combined, then sprinkle over the hazelnuts.

Often the simplest dishes are the best, yet quality, season and the ripeness of the tomatoes are key to the success of this one. Lemon thyme is a personal favourite, but basil, oregano or chives would also work well here.

heritage tomatoes with lemon thyme

600 g/1lb 5 oz. ripe
  heritage tomatoes in
  various colours,
  shapes and sizes, at
  room temperature
fruity extra virgin olive
  oil, for drizzling

2–3 tablespoons lemon
  thyme or basil leaves
sea salt

Serves 4

Halve, quarter or leave the tomatoes whole, depending on their size and shape.

Arrange on a serving platter and drizzle with olive oil. Season with salt and sprinkle the lemon thyme over. Serve at room temperature.

BRUSSELS SPROUTS

Whether lightly cooked or served raw, Brussels sprouts go particularly well with salty or nutty flavoured ingredients, such as bacon, ham, grains, walnuts or hazelnuts, as here.

TOMATOES

Heritage, or heirloom, tomatoes come in a wide range of colours, shapes and sizes and their diversity is the beauty of this salad.

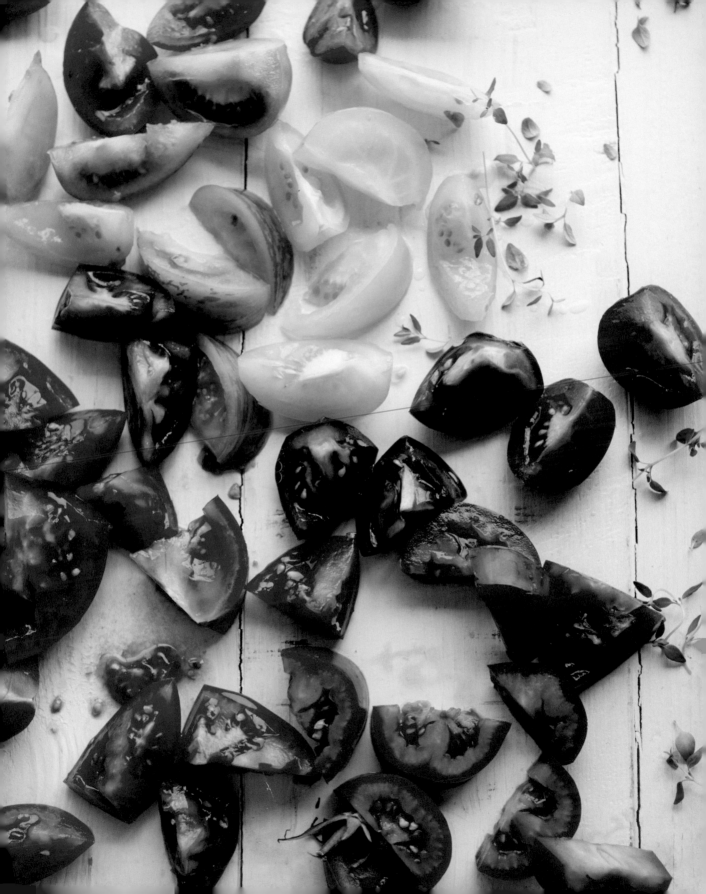

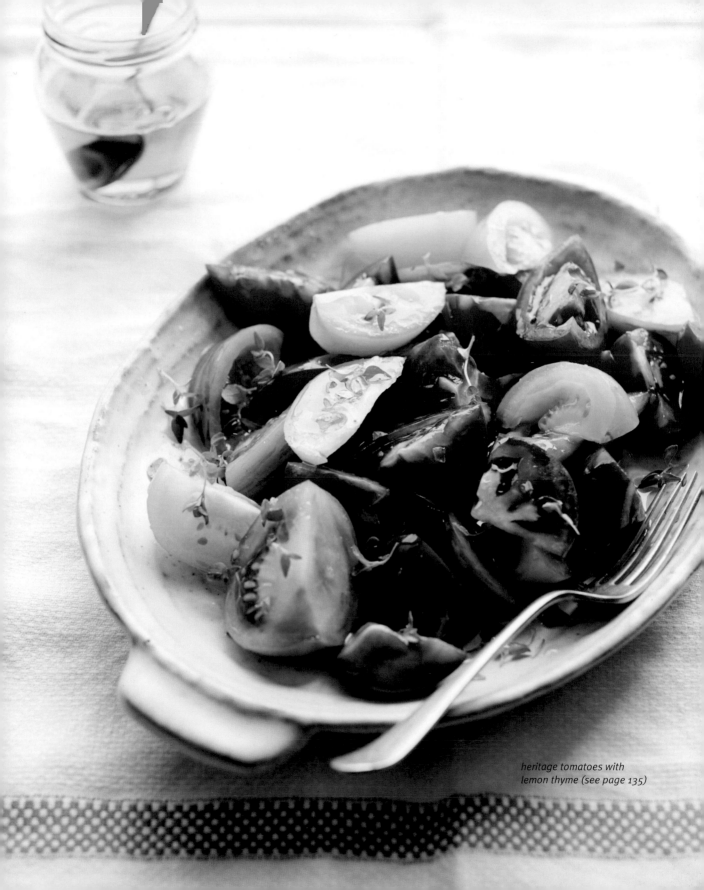

heritage tomatoes with
lemon thyme (see page 135)

Make the most of the short asparagus season with this deliciously simple and easy salad. The slightly charred spears are drizzled with a light, fragrant herb oil instead of the more usual mayonnaise or hollandaise sauce.

char-grilled asparagus with herb oil

300 g/11 oz. asparagus
  spears, ends trimmed
HERB OIL
3 tablespoons extra
  virgin olive oil, plus
  extra for brushing
a large handful of mixed
  finely chopped herbs,
  such as basil, oregano
  and thyme

1 small garlic clove,
  crushed
freshly squeezed juice
  of ½ lemon
sea salt and freshly
  ground black pepper

Serves 4

To make the herb oil, mix together all the ingredients in a bowl and season to taste. Set aside while you griddle the asparagus.

Heat a large, ridged griddle pan over a high heat. Brush the asparagus spears with oil and season. Griddle the asparagus, in two batches, for 5–8 minutes, turning them occasionally, or until tender and slightly charred in places. Serve the asparagus drizzled with the herb oil.

The lemon-mustard dressing enlivens the stems of lightly steamed broccoli in this easy side salad. It goes well with fish, lamb and chicken dishes. If you can't find long-stem broccoli, use regular broccoli instead.

long-stem broccoli with lemon-mustard dressing

400 g/14 oz. long-stem
  broccoli, trimmed
a small handful of radish
  sprouts (optional)
**LEMON-MUSTARD
DRESSING**
3 tablespoons extra
  virgin olive oil

1 garlic clove, finely
  chopped
2 tablespoons freshly
  squeezed lemon juice
1 teaspoon Dijon mustard
sea salt and freshly
  ground black pepper

Serves 4

Steam the broccoli for 2–3 minutes until only just tender, then refresh under cold running water to prevent it cooking any further and to keep its colour. Drain.

Meanwhile, make the dressing. Heat the oil and garlic in a small pan over a low heat for 1 minute, then stir in the lemon juice and mustard, season and warm through briefly.

Arrange the broccoli on a serving plate, spoon the dressing over and sprinkle the radish sprouts on top, if using.

SPROUTING BROCCOLI
Grown with either green or purple coloured florets, for the best flavour opt for tightly packed broccoli heads with firm stems.

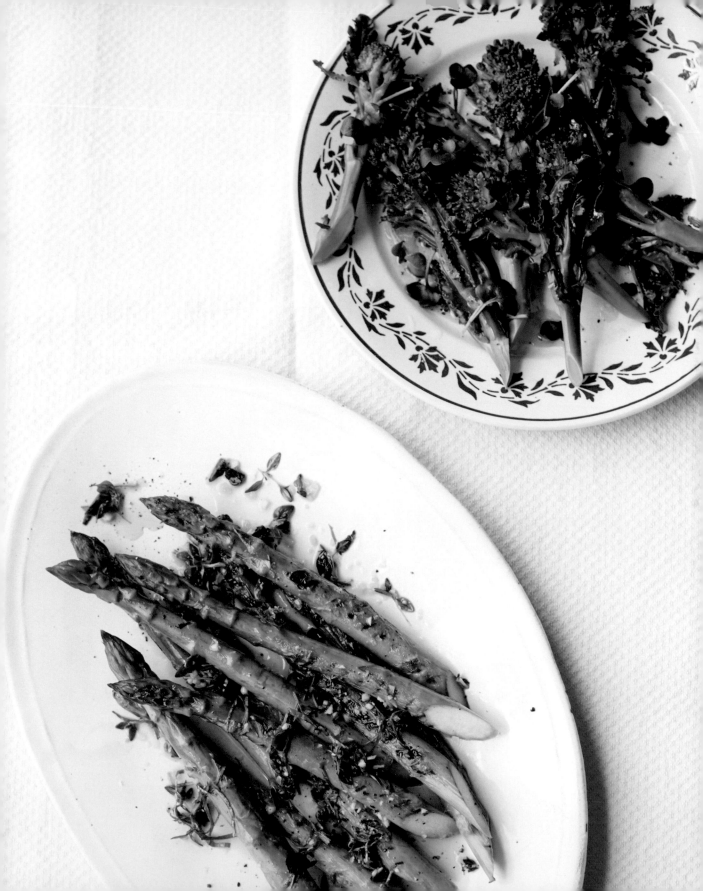

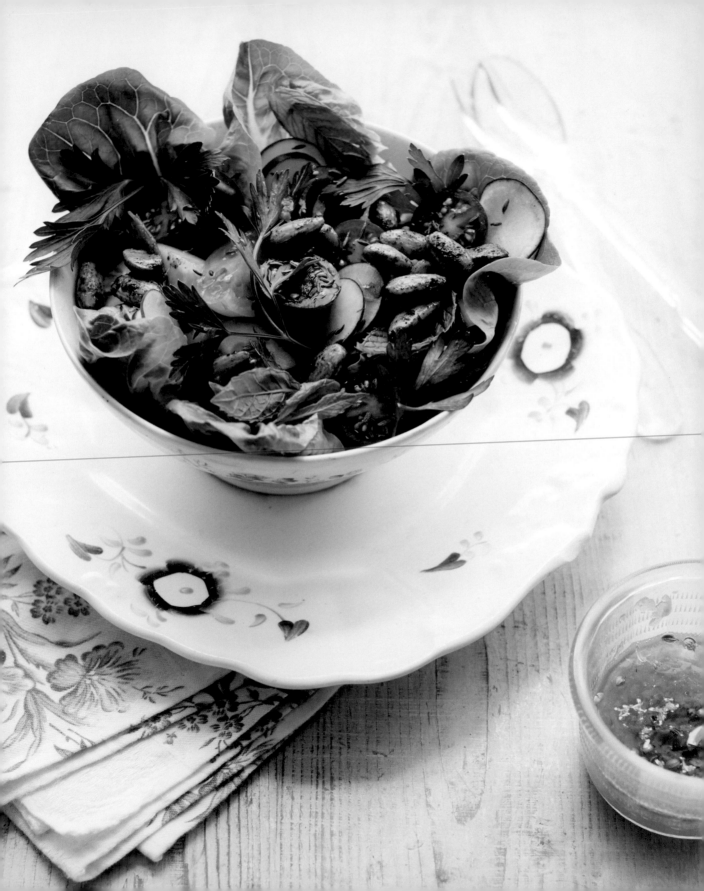

This twist on the popular Lebanese salad is made with vibrant, crisp vegetables in an orangey pistachio oil dressing. Instead of the more usual addition of crisp toasted pitta bread, the salad is topped with smoked paprika roasted almonds. If you can't find pistachio oil, simply increase the quantity of olive oil.

fattoush with spiced almonds

1 tablespoon smoked
    hot paprika
60 g/½ cup blanched
    almonds
2 small Little Gem/Bibb
    lettuces, leaves
    separated
250 g/9 oz. vine-ripened
    cherry tomatoes,
    halved
1 small Lebanese
    cucumber, quartered
    lengthways and cut
    into bite-sized chunks
1 large romano or red
    (bell) pepper, seeded
    and cut into bite-sized
    chunks
8 radishes, sliced
    into rounds
5 tablespoons freshly
    chopped mint leaves
5 tablespoons freshly
    chopped parsley
    leaves
½ teaspoon cumin seeds,
    toasted
sea salt and freshly
    ground black pepper

ORANGE & PISTACHIO DRESSING
3 tablespoons extra
    virgin olive oil
3 tablespoons
    pistachio oil
finely grated zest and
    freshly squeezed juice
    of 1 small orange
1 teaspoon coriander
    seeds, toasted and
    ground

Serves 4

Preheat the oven to 180°C (350°F) Gas 4.

Mix together the paprika and 1 tablespoon of the olive oil in a bowl, season and add the almonds. Turn to coat the almonds in the paprika oil and shake onto a baking sheet. Spread the nuts out evenly and roast in the preheated oven for 15–20 minutes, turning once, until they start to turn golden. Leave to cool.

Meanwhile, make the orange and pistachio dressing. Put all the ingredients in a small jar, season, and shake until combined.

Arrange the Little Gem/Bibb lettuce leaves on a large serving platter and top with the tomatoes, cucumber, red (bell) pepper, radishes, mint and parsley. Spoon the dressing over the salad and toss gently until combined. Sprinkle with cumin seeds and the almonds before serving.

PISTACHIO OIL

Pressed from pistachios, this nut oil has a wonderful vibrant green colour and intensely nutty flavour. Since nut oils can be quite strong in flavour, they should be used judiciously or tempered by mixing with a mild-tasting oil. They also work well with sweet ingredients, such as fruit or honey.

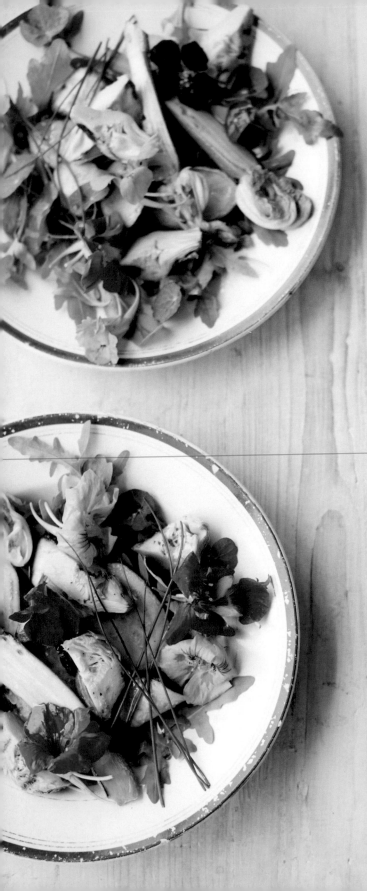

It's easy to forget to use flowers in food, but edible ones naturally lend themselves to salads, adding both colour and flavour. Here, courgette/zucchini, nasturtium and chive flowers are used, but feel free to experiment with others such as borage, marigolds, violas and pansies. Do make sure that the flowers have been grown organically and check that they are edible before use.

shoots, flowers & leaves

2 tablespoons extra virgin olive oil, plus extra for drizzling
1 yellow courgette/ zucchini, sliced diagonally, plus flower, halved, if available
1 green courgette/ zucchini, sliced diagonally, plus flower, halved, if available
100 g/3¾ oz. rocket/ arugula leaves
180 g/6 oz. char-grilled artichokes

a handful of small nasturtium leaves
10 chive stems, snipped (with flowers if possible)
1 tablespoon lemon thyme leaves
freshly squeezed juice of ½ lemon
8 nasturtium flowers
sea salt and freshly ground black pepper

Serves 4

Heat the olive oil in a large frying pan/skillet over a medium heat and sauté the sliced courgettes/zucchini for 5 minutes, turning once, until tender and slightly golden. Leave to cool slightly.

Put the rocket/arugula on a serving plate and top with the courgettes/zucchini, artichokes, nasturtium leaves, snipped chives and lemon thyme. Squeeze over the lemon juice and drizzle with a little extra olive oil. Season and toss gently until combined.

Just before serving, garnish with the flowers.

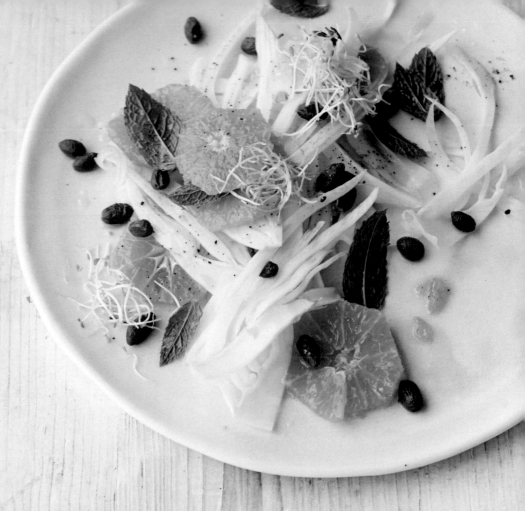

Light, refreshing and vibrant, this salad goes particularly well with baked or grilled/broiled fish. Make this salad just before serving to retain its freshness.

fennel, clementine & alfalfa salad

2 tablespoons dried goji
    berries
2 fennel bulbs, trimmed,
    fronds reserved and
    bulbs thinly sliced
2 clementines, peeled,
    pith removed, and
    sliced into rounds
2 handfuls of alfalfa
    sprouts
2 tablespoons fresh
    mint leaves

DRESSING
4 tablespoons extra
    virgin olive oil
4 teaspoons white wine
    vinegar
sea salt and freshly
    ground black pepper

Serves 4

Soak the goji berries in just-boiled water for 5 minutes until softened, then drain.

Meanwhile, mix together all the ingredients for the dressing and season.

Arrange the fennel, clementines and alfalfa sprouts on a serving plate. Sprinkle with the goji berries and spoon the dressing over the top. Garnish with fennel fronds and mint.

Make the most of summer vegetables when in season with this pretty, vibrant side salad. The herb-infused home-made mayonnaise adds the final flourish! This is delicious served with fresh crab or poached salmon and buttered new potatoes. Do opt for frozen peas and beans if fresh ones are out of season.

summer vegetable salad with herb mayonnaise

300 g/11 oz. shelled
  broad/fava beans
200 g/7 oz. shelled
  fresh peas
200 g/7 oz. asparagus
  spears, trimmed
200 g/7 oz. baby
  courgettes/zucchini,
  halved lengthways
1 tablespoon extra virgin
  olive oil
sea salt and freshly
  ground black pepper

HERB MAYONNAISE
6 tablespoons
  mayonnaise
  (see page 12)
3 tablespoons freshly
  squeezed lemon juice
2 tablespoons freshly
  snipped chives
2 tablespoons freshly
  snipped dill
1 small garlic clove,
  crushed

Serves 4

Steam the broad/fava beans and peas for 2–3 minutes until tender, then refresh under cold running water. Slip the beans out of their grey outer shells and put in a serving bowl with the peas.

Steam the asparagus for 3 minutes or until tender, then refresh under cold running water. Slice the stems of the asparagus, leaving about 3 cm/1 in. of the head intact, then add to the bowl. Pour the olive oil into the bowl, season, and toss until everything is combined.

To make the herb mayonnaise, mix together the mayonnaise, lemon juice, herbs and garlic in a bowl, adding a spoonful or two of water to loosen slightly, if needed. Serve the vegetables topped with a spoonful of the herb mayonnaise.

The spice mix togarashi is a punchy, aromatic combination of chilli/chile, orange, ginger and Szechuan pepper, but it is optional here, so don't worry if you can't get hold of it.

char-grilled aubergines with miso dressing

2 aubergines/eggplants
3 tablespoons sesame oil
3 tablespoons cold-
  pressed rapeseed oil
2 teaspoons toasted
  sesame seeds
togarashi spice mix, for
  sprinkling (optional)
1 spring onion/scallion,
  shredded, to serve

MISO DRESSING
2 tablespoons yellow
  miso paste
2 tablespoons light soy
  sauce
2 tablespoons mirin
1 tablespoon maple syrup
2.5-cm/1-in. piece fresh
  root ginger, peeled
  and grated

Serves 4

Cut the aubergines/eggplants into thin slices lengthways, discarding the two outermost slices. Heat a large, ridged griddle pan over a high heat. Mix together the sesame oil and rapeseed oil and brush some over one side of the aubergine/eggplant slices. Griddle the aubergine/eggplant slices, in batches, for 10–12 minutes, turning once until tender and charred in places. Brush with extra oil when you turn them over.

Meanwhile, to make the dressing, mix together the miso paste, soy sauce, mirin and maple syrup. Squeeze the ginger in one hand to extract the juice and add the juice to the dressing. Stir well until combined.

Transfer the aubergine/eggplant slices to a serving plate and spoon enough of the miso dressing over to coat. Sprinkle with the sesame seeds, togarashi, if using, and shredded spring onion/scallion.

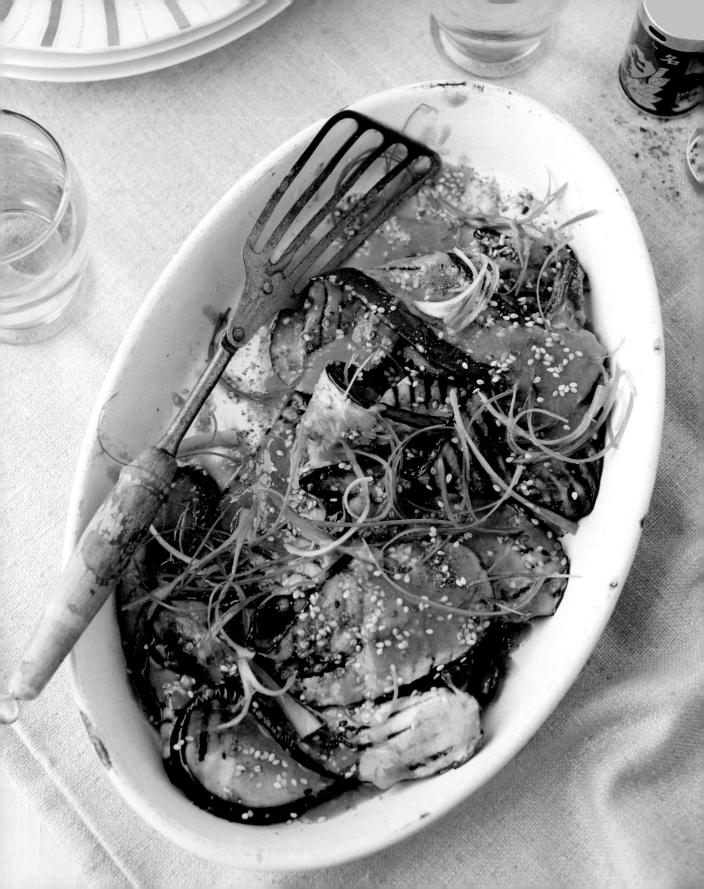

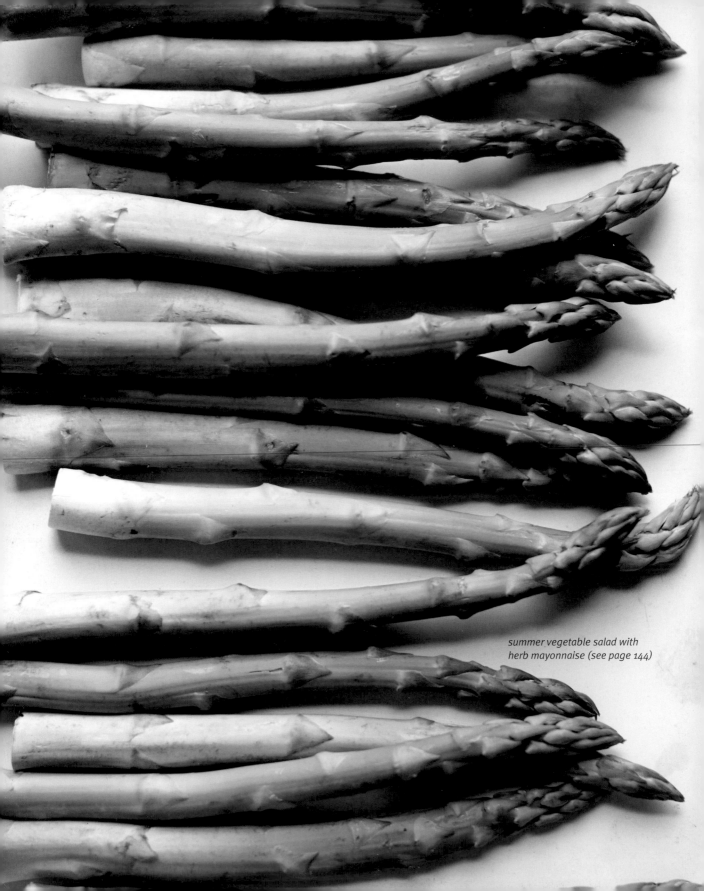

summer vegetable salad with
herb mayonnaise (see page 144)

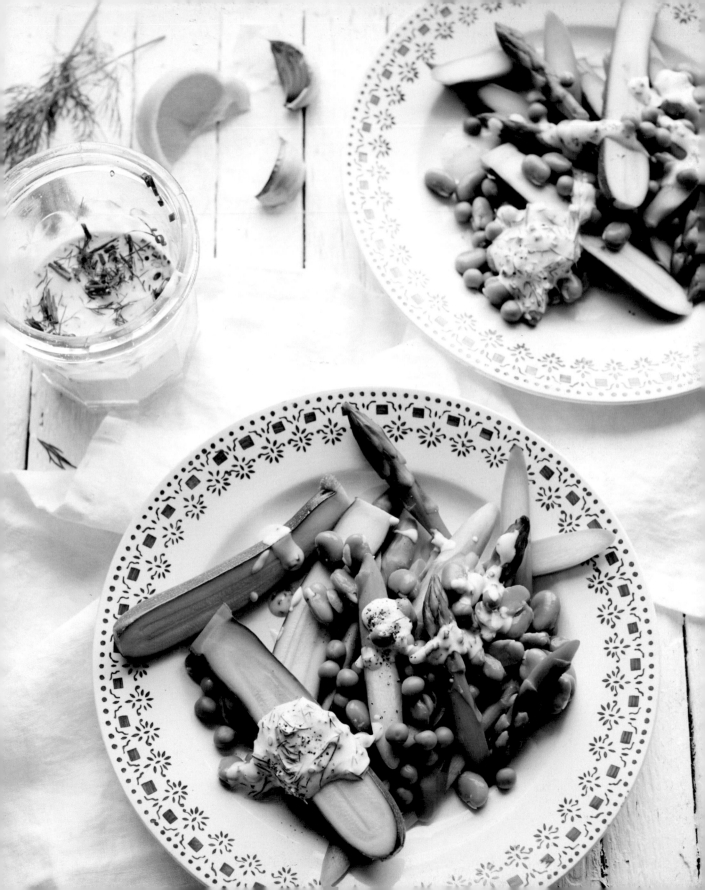

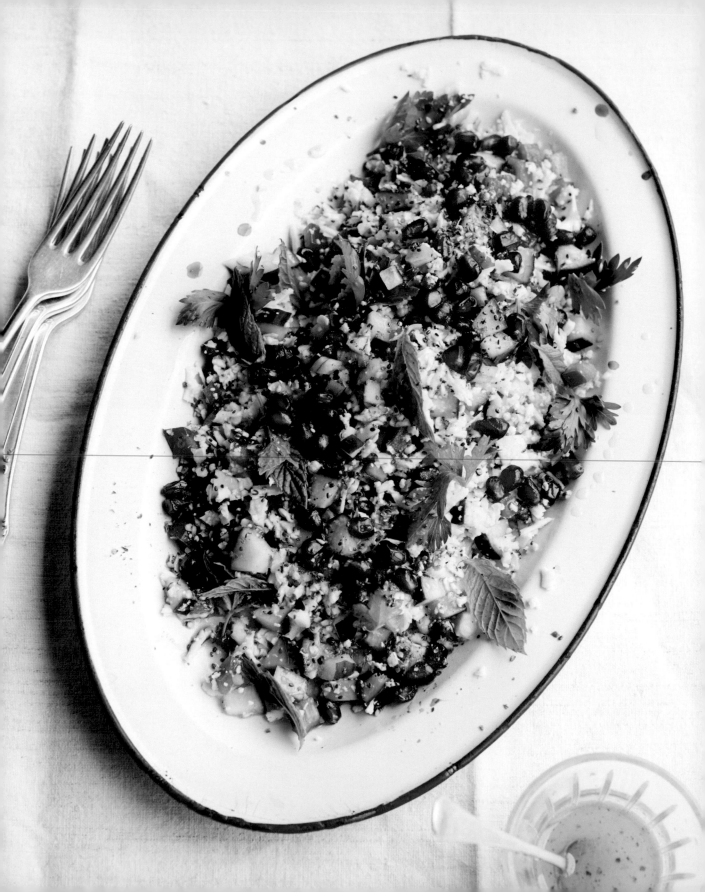

Cauliflower, when grated into fine grains, makes a surprisingly good and nutritious alternative to couscous, and is both low-carbohydrate and gluten-free. Pomegranate and chia seeds boost the nutritional status of this pretty and vibrant salad even further. Serve it as a light meal or as part of a mezze selection.

cauliflower couscous with pomegranate

1 cauliflower, leaves removed
1 small red onion, diced
1 small cucumber, quartered lengthways, seeded and diced
1 red (bell) pepper, seeded and diced
2 large handfuls of freshly chopped mint leaves
2 large handfuls of freshly chopped flat leaf parsley
seeds from ¼–½ pomegranate, depending on size

1 teaspoon chia seeds (optional)
2 teaspoons za'atar (see page 11)

DRESSING
5 tablespoons extra virgin olive oil
finely grated zest of ½ lemon
freshly squeezed juice of 1 lemon
sea salt and freshly ground black pepper

Serves 4

Mix together all the ingredients for the dressing, season and set aside.

Grate the cauliflower florets into fine "grains" using the large holes of a box grater and discard the stalks (these can be used in another dish). Put the cauliflower into a shallow serving bowl and top with the red onion, cucumber, red (bell) pepper, mint, parsley, pomegranate seeds and chia seeds, if using.

Spoon the dressing over the salad and turn until it is coated and everything is combined. Serve, sprinkled with za'atar.

CHIA SEEDS
These tiny black seeds are said to be one of the richest plant sources of omega-3 fatty acids. They become gelatinous when soaked in water, which is said to increase bioavailability, although this is unnecessary if using in small quantities.

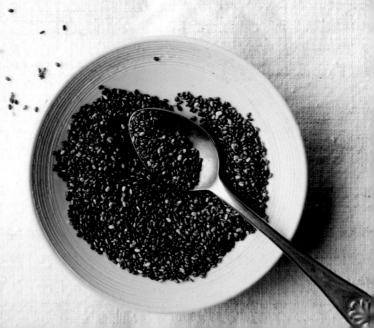

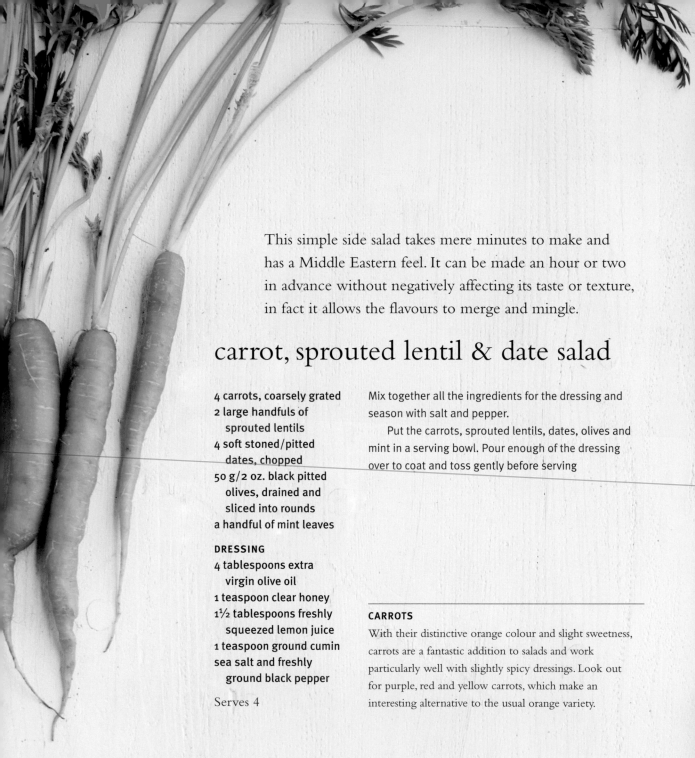

This simple side salad takes mere minutes to make and has a Middle Eastern feel. It can be made an hour or two in advance without negatively affecting its taste or texture, in fact it allows the flavours to merge and mingle.

carrot, sprouted lentil & date salad

4 carrots, coarsely grated
2 large handfuls of
 sprouted lentils
4 soft stoned/pitted
 dates, chopped
50 g/2 oz. black pitted
 olives, drained and
 sliced into rounds
a handful of mint leaves

DRESSING
4 tablespoons extra
 virgin olive oil
1 teaspoon clear honey
1½ tablespoons freshly
 squeezed lemon juice
1 teaspoon ground cumin
sea salt and freshly
 ground black pepper

Serves 4

Mix together all the ingredients for the dressing and season with salt and pepper.

Put the carrots, sprouted lentils, dates, olives and mint in a serving bowl. Pour enough of the dressing over to coat and toss gently before serving

CARROTS

With their distinctive orange colour and slight sweetness, carrots are a fantastic addition to salads and work particularly well with slightly spicy dressings. Look out for purple, red and yellow carrots, which make an interesting alternative to the usual orange variety.

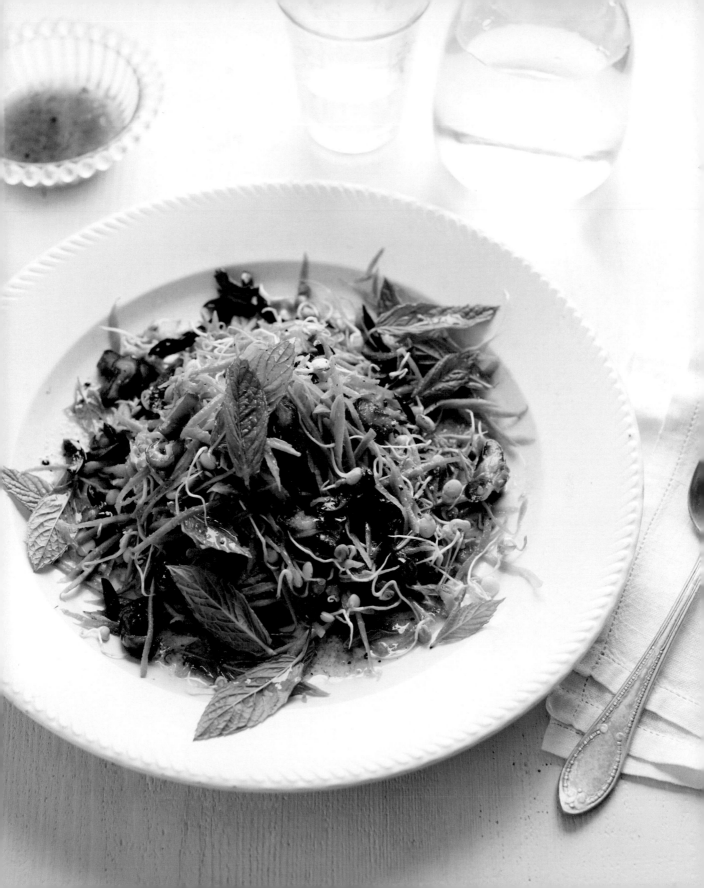

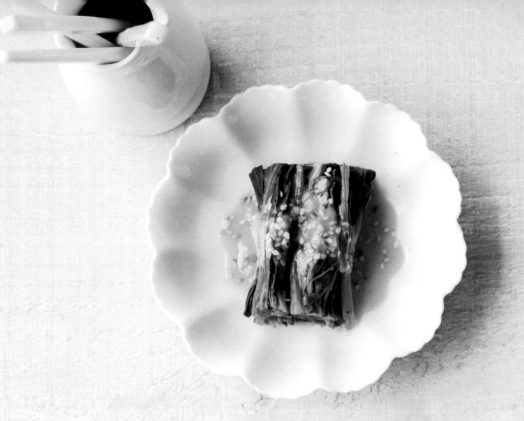

A Japanese-inspired salad, which is simplicity itself… Tahini, the sesame seed paste, lends a nutritious, nutty creaminess to the dressing. This would also be delicious spooned over steamed asparagus, edamame beans or fine green beans.

spinach with tahini dressing

400 g/14 oz. spinach
  leaves, tough stalks
  removed
2 teaspoons toasted
  sesame seeds

TAHINI DRESSING
1 tablespoon sunflower
  oil
2 garlic cloves, sliced
4 tablespoons mirin
2 heaped tablespoons
  light tahini
1 tablespoon toasted
  sesame oil

Serves 4

To make the tahini dressing, heat the oil and garlic in a small pan over a low heat for 1 minute or until the garlic loses its pungency. Put the garlic and oil into a bowl and stir in the mirin, tahini and sesame oil. Stir until combined, adding a splash of water if needed to make a dressing the consistency of single/light cream.

Meanwhile, steam the spinach for 3 minutes until the leaves have just wilted. (Use tongs to turn the leaves occasionally in the steamer so they cook evenly.) Drain and transfer the spinach to a shallow serving bowl. Spoon the dressing over and sprinkle with sesame seeds. Serve warm or at room temperature.

If you have a spiralizer, a utensil that allows you to slice vegetables into thin "noodles", then this salad is perfect for you.

hijiki & vegetable "noodles"

17 g/½ oz. dried hijiki
1 carrot, halved crossways
1 small cucumber, quartered lengthways, and seeded
1 red (bell) pepper, seeded
14 cm/5½ in. piece daikon/mooli, peeled and halved
2 tablespoons pumpkin seeds, toasted
2 tablespoons pink pickled ginger
2 tablespoons shiso sprouts or radish sprouts

DRESSING
1 tablespoon sesame oil
3 tablespoons rice wine vinegar
2 tablespoons mirin
2 tablespoons tamari or light soy sauce
2 teaspoons very finely chopped fresh root ginger
freshly ground black pepper

Serves 4

Soak the hijiki in plenty of cold water for 10 minutes until softened. Drain, rinse and transfer to a pan. Cover with fresh cold water, bring almost to the boil, then turn the heat down and simmer for 10 minutes until tender. Drain and refresh under cold running water.

Meanwhile, mix together all the ingredients for the dressing, season with pepper and set aside.

Slice the carrot, cucumber, red (bell) pepper and daikon/mooli into long, thin strips and put in a serving dish with the hijiki. Spoon enough of the dressing over to coat and toss gently until combined. Sprinkle with the pumpkin seeds and top with a pile of pink pickled ginger and shiso sprouts.

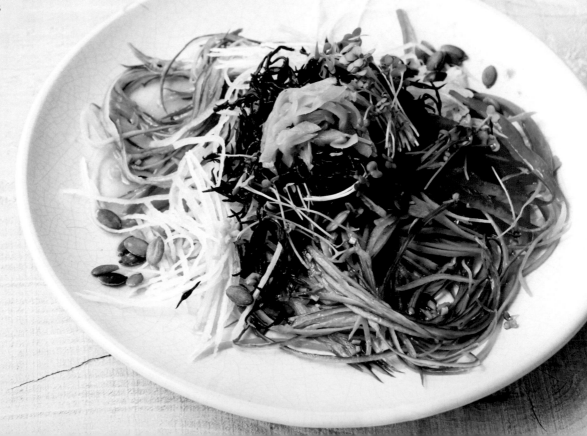

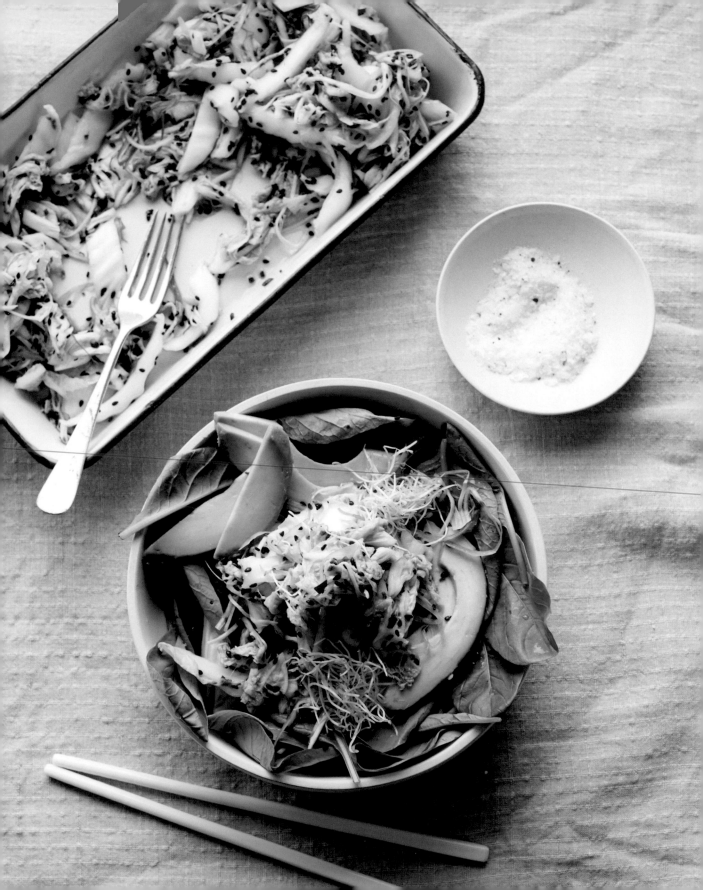

Kimchi, the highly popular Korean pickle, traditionally takes a few days to make and ferment, but with this 'cheats' version, it needs a comparatively short amount of time, just enough to let the flavours meld and mingle.

kimchi, avocado & alfalfa salad

2 Chinese leaves/
  Chinese cabbage,
  shredded
2 spring onions/
  scallions, shredded
1 red chilli/chile,
  seeded and diced
2.5-cm/1-in. piece fresh
  root ginger, peeled and
  very thinly sliced
2 tablespoons black
  sesame seeds, toasted
4 tablespoons rice
  vinegar

4 teaspoons caster/
  superfine sugar
½ teaspoon sea salt
2 tablespoons cold-
  pressed rapeseed oil
75 g/3 oz. baby spinach
  leaves
2 avocados, halved,
  stoned/pitted, peeled
  and sliced
2 handfuls of alfalfa
  sprouts

Serves 4

First make the kimchi. Mix together the Chinese leaves/Chinese cabbage, spring onions/scallions, chilli/chile, ginger, sesame seeds, rice vinegar, caster/superfine sugar and salt in a bowl and leave to sit for 30 minutes (or longer if time allows) to let the flavours develop.

Just before serving, divide the spinach and avocados between 4 serving plates, drizzle with the oil and top with the kimchi and alfalfa sprouts.

A refreshing change to the more usual mayonnaise-coated coleslaw, this version has a zingy sesame and ginger dressing. Experiment with different combinations of vegetables such as white cabbage, kale and Brussels sprouts, or include fruit such as apples or pears.

Asian slaw

200 g/7 oz. red cabbage,
  shredded
8 cm/3 in. piece daikon/
  mooli, peeled and
  grated
2 carrots, grated
4 spring onions/
  scallions, thinly sliced
5 tablespoons of torn
  Thai basil leaves

SESAME GINGER
DRESSING
2 tablespoons sesame oil
2 tablespoons cold-
  pressed rapeseed oil
2 tablespoons rice
  vinegar
2.5-cm/1-in. piece fresh
  root ginger, peeled
  and grated
sea salt and freshly
  ground black pepper

Serves 4

To make the dressing, mix together the sesame oil, rapeseed oil and rice vinegar. Squeeze the ginger in one hand to extract the juice and add to the dressing, then season.

Put the red cabbage, daikon/mooli, carrots, spring onions/scallions and basil in a serving bowl. Add the dressing and toss the salad until well combined. Serve at room temperature.

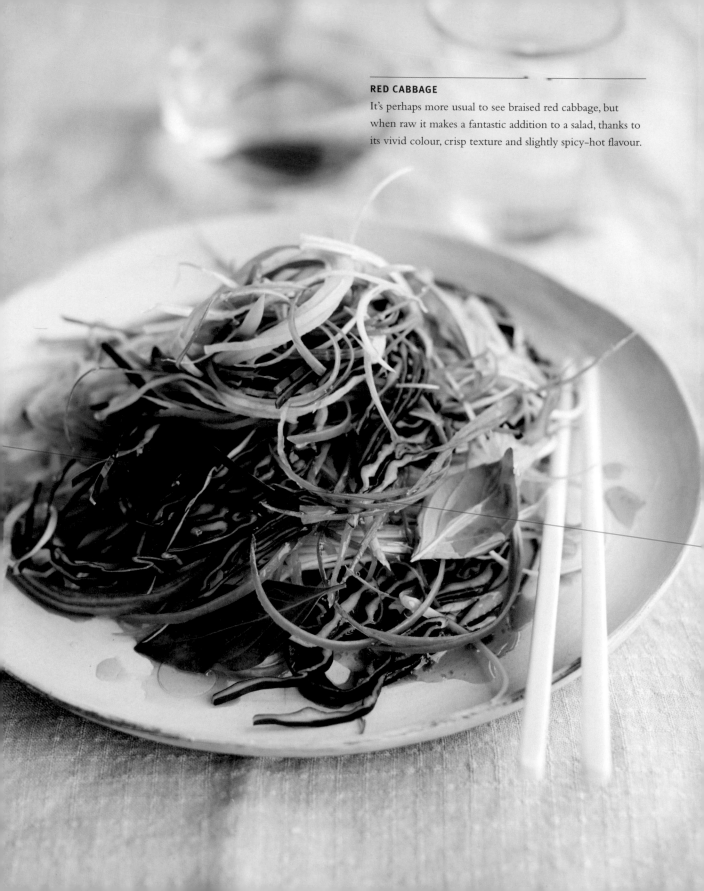

RED CABBAGE
It's perhaps more usual to see braised red cabbage, but when raw it makes a fantastic addition to a salad, thanks to its vivid colour, crisp texture and slightly spicy–hot flavour.

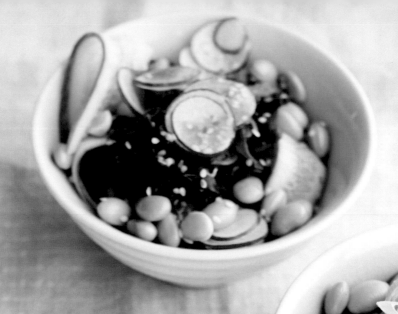

Wakame is popular in miso soup, but this sea vegetable also makes a great addition to Japanese-style salads. It is mild and slightly sweet in taste, with a subtle saltiness reminiscent of the sea.

Japanese wakame, radish & edamame salad

50 g/2 oz. frozen
   edamame beans
12 g/½ oz. dried wakame
   seaweed, rinsed
½ small cucumber, sliced
   into ribbons
115 g/4 oz. radishes,
   thinly sliced into
   rounds
70 g/3 oz. sugar snap
   peas, trimmed and
   sliced diagonally
2 spring onions/
   scallions, thinly sliced
   diagonally
2 teaspoons toasted
   sesame seeds

DRESSING
2 tablespoons sunflower
   oil
1 tablespoon sesame oil
2 tablespoons rice wine
   vinegar
1 tablespoon light soy
   sauce

Serves 4

Steam the edamame beans for 2–3 minutes until tender, then refresh under cold running water and drain.

Meanwhile, put the wakame in a bowl, pour over enough cold water to cover and leave to soak for 3 minutes until rehydrated, then drain.

Mix together all the ingredients for the dressing in a small bowl.

Put the cucumber in a large, shallow serving bowl with the cooked edamame beans, soaked wakame, radishes, sugar snap peas and spring onions/scallions. Spoon the dressing over and toss the salad until evenly coated. Sprinkle the sesame seeds over before serving.

index

acknowledgments

This has been such a lovely, enjoyable book to write and all made possible thanks to the team at RPS. My heartfelt thanks, as always, go to editorial director, Julia Charles, for commissioning me to write this book. I would also like to say a big thank you to publisher, Cindy Richards; Kate Eddison, who calmly and efficiently worked on the text; designer Megan Smith; photographer Matt Russell, for his wonderful, inspirational shots; food stylists Aya Nishimura and Xenia Von Oswald for making my recipes look so appetizing; and prop stylist, Jo Harris.

ABOUT THE AUTHOR

Nicola Graimes is an award-winning writer specializing in nutritional health, vegetarian cooking, and food for children. A former editor of Vegetarian Living magazine, she has written more than 26 books, including *Great Healthy Food for Vegetarian Kids*, which won Best Vegetarian Cookbook in the World Gourmand Awards 2010. For Ryland Peters & Small she has written *Super Fresh Juices & Smoothies*.

ABOUT THE PHOTOGRAPHER

Matt Russell is a London-based photographer specializing in food, travel, lifestyle and portraiture. With a strong reputation for his natural style and ability to capture life, Matt has established himself internationally as a trusted, reputable photographer.

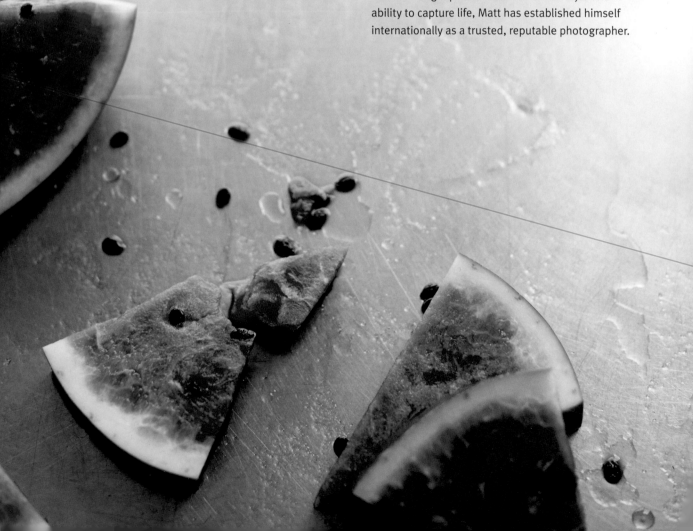